Praise for Pilates For Dummies

"This book is extraordinary as it provides detailed information on the Pilates concepts and applies them to other modalities such as the ball and roller. Ms. Herman stresses stretching and strengthening, a point which many other programs lack."

— Erica Essner, Pilates trainer, The Method

"The pregnant woman finally has exercise guidelines that make sense for her body. Ms. Herman has tremendous insight into the pregnant and post-natal body and gives excellent recommendations for keeping a woman's reproducing body toned and happy."

— Gail Herrine, MD, Obstetrician/Gynecologist

"For the last decade we've been hearing about how Pilates is transforming the bodies of the rich and famous. Now at last there's a Pilates bible for the rest of us. With careful attention to detail and an irreverent sense of humor, Ellie Herman untangles the pretzel of Pilates and shows how it truly can offer a fitness program for everyone. The result is not just a how-to book, but a deeply persuasive tract on how exercising the body intelligently can heal injuries, reform posture, and give you a new lease on life."

— Carol Lloyd, author of *Creating a Life Worth Living*

"For those of us who want movie-star bodies but can't afford a personal trainer, *Pilates For Dummies* is the quickest, simplest, and most entertaining book you'll find for firming your flesh forever. Ellie Herman not only knows her Pilates, she also knows how to write with the same grace, punch, and power you'll develop after practicing the exercises in this little gem of a book."

— Sylvia Paull, former book reviewer, *Wired* magazine, bicycle racer, and Pilates practitioner

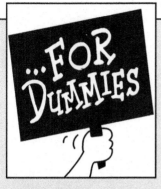
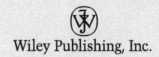

Pilates
FOR
DUMMIES®

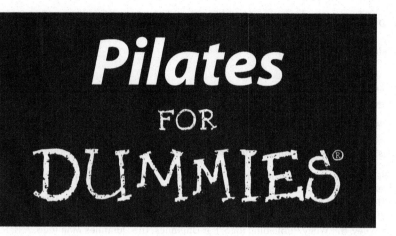

Pilates FOR DUMMIES®

by Ellie Herman

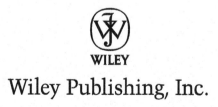

WILEY

Wiley Publishing, Inc.

Pilates For Dummies®

Published by
Wiley Publishing, Inc.
111 River St.
Hoboken, NJ 07030
www.wiley.com

Copyright © 2002 by Wiley Publishing, Inc., Indianapolis, Indiana

Published simultaneously in Canada

For general information on our other products and services or to obtain technical support, please contact our Customer Care Department within the U.S. at 800-762-2974, outside the U.S. at 317-572-3993, or fax 317-572-4002.

Wiley also publishes its books in a variety of electronic formats. Some content that appears in print may not be available in electronic books.

Library of Congress Control Number: 2002100169

ISBN: 978-0-7645-5397-4

10 9 8

1O/TR/RQ/QX/IN

WILEY

About the Author

Ellie Herman, M.S., LAc, runs two thriving Pilates studios, one in San Francisco and one in Oakland. The Ellie Herman Studios offer annual teacher training intensives in Northern California. Ellie has certified instructors locally, nationally, and internationally. She has taught Pilates for over ten years and has developed a unique language to communicate the essence of the Pilates method. She was first introduced to Pilates in 1988 as a rehabilitation patient at Saint Francis Hospital Dance Medicine in San Francisco. She received her formal Pilates training in 1991 in New York City, where she studied with two of the original Pilates protégés, Romana Kryzanowska and Kathy Grant.

Formerly a professional dancer and choreographer with her own dance company, Ellie has a background that includes contemporary dance techniques, yoga, gymnastics, kinesiology, and anatomy. She is a licensed acupuncturist with a Master of Science degree in acupuncture and Chinese herbal medicine. In her studios, Ellie combines Pilates with acupuncture and body work to offer a complete rehabilitation and wellness environment. Ellie strives to integrate her studies and continually expand her approach to bring balance back to the body. (Check out Chapter 4 for photos of Ellie in action.)

Author's Acknowledgments

I would like to acknowledge all of my teachers who ever taught me anything about the body, including many of my students. To name a few: Kathy Grant, Jennifer Stacey, Romana Kyrzanowska, Steve Giordano, Jayne Edwards, and Cara Reeser.

I would also like to thank all the beautiful models, who are mostly instructors at my studios: Carie Lee (beginning series), Caleb Rhodes (intermediate series), Sharon Gallagher (advanced series), Jessica Fudim (big ball), Janine Fondiller (roller and posture photos), Sarah Khalouf (small ball), Valeria Russell (the wall), Louise Laub-Goodrich (pregnancy), Martina Nevermann (pregnancy, and also thanks for the costumes!)

I would also like to thank my brother, David Herman, for taking the gorgeous photos and Jordan for doing the fabulous lighting! Thanks to Walt and Nancy Herman for babysitting so Dave and Martina could do the photo shoot. Thanks to Susi May for being the technical editor and a wonderful instructor. Thanks to all the other instructors and support staff at the studio for working hard while the author was at home writing: Lizz Roman, Melissa Harrington, Donna Rosen, Jenna Marshall, Lise Pruitt, Becca Wieder, Jaime Michel, Kate Thorngren, Nicole Dessoye, Chris Black, Marcelle Parry, Linda XYZ, Angelina Vasile, and Kristin Iuppenlatz. Thanks, Monique, for moving your yoga class during the photo shoot. Thanks to Phil Cusick for always being there. Thanks to Carol Lloyd for her inspiration to really enjoy the process of writing and to make the subject sizzle. Thanks to my agent, Jayne Rockmill, for making it all possible.

Publisher's Acknowledgments

We're proud of this book; please send us your comments through our Dummies online registration form located at www.dummies.com/register/.

Some of the people who helped bring this book to market include the following:

Acquisitions, Editorial, and Media Development

Associate Project Editor: Ben Nussbaum

Acquisitions Editors: Stacy S. Collins, Kevin Thornton

Senior Copy Editors: Tina Sims, Patricia Yuu Pan

Technical Editor: Susi May

Editorial Managers: Pam Mourouzis, Christine Meloy Beck

Editorial Assistants: Melissa Bennett, Nívea C. Strickland

Photo Credits: David Herman, Jordan Levy

Cover Photo: David Herman and Jordan Levy

Composition Services

Project Coordinator: Jennifer Bingham

Layout and Graphics: Beth Brooks, Jackie Nicholas, Julie Trippetti, Jeremey Unger, Mary J. Virgin

Proofreaders: John Greenough, Betty Kish, Carl Pierce, Linda Quigley

Indexer: Liz Cunningham

Publishing and Editorial for Consumer Dummies

Diane Graves Steele, Vice President and Publisher, Consumer Dummies

Joyce Pepple, Acquisitions Director, Consumer Dummies

Kristin A. Cocks, Product Development Director, Consumer Dummies

Michael Spring, Vice President and Publisher, Travel

Brice Gosnell, Associate Publisher, Travel

Suzanne Jannetta, Editorial Director, Travel

Publishing for Technology Dummies

Andy Cummings, Vice President and Publisher, Dummies Technology/General User

Composition Services

Gerry Fahey, Vice President of Production Services

Debbie Stailey, Director of Composition Services

Contents at a Glance

Cartoons at a Glance

By Rich Tennant

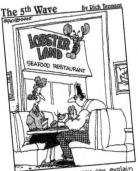

page 5

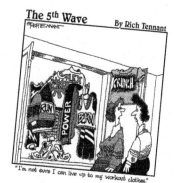

page 43

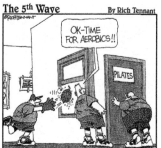

page 203

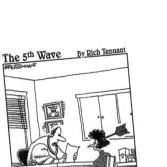

page 267

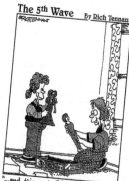

page 293

Cartoon Information:
Fax: 978-546-7747
E-Mail: richtennant@the5thwave.com
World Wide Web: www.the5thwave.com

Table of Contents

Chapter 6: Feeling Stronger Every Day: Intermediate Mat Exercises 87

Chapter 7: More Than a Washboard: The Advanced Mat Series 113

Introduction

●●●

*P*ilates has become one of the most popular fitness methods in the
United States. Every other Hollywood star seems to be doing it, and
Pilates mat classes are offered at almost every gym in every small town
around the country. This book is primarily meant to give you a comprehen-
sive overview of the Pilates mat workout. In addition, I include lots of information about the background, history, and philosophy underlying the Pilates
method. If you want to go beyond the mat, you also can find information
about Pilates equipment and accessories and special programs for the pregnant, the elderly, and the injured.

About This Book

You can read every *For Dummies* book straight through, from the first to the
last chapter. Or, you can browse through it, flipping to chapters that you find
especially interesting. But given that Pilates is a discipline in which you really
get better gradually, you probably don't want to jump straight into the complicated exercises.

You can use this book in several ways:

- ✔ If you're a novice, you probably want to start right here in the Introduction
  and then read Part I, which contains the first three chapters. Then introduce yourself to Pilates by doing the mat series in Chapter 4. If you want,
  you can then skip ahead to Chapters 11 through 14, which contain exercises using Pilates accessories that you can add to your routine. If you're
  new to Pilates, I recommend that you stay away from the more advanced
  exercises until you have some experience with the basic movements and
  have given yourself a chance to build your strength and increase your
  flexibility.

- ✔ If you already know a lot about Pilates and are just looking for a few more
  exercises to add to your routine, flip through Chapters 4 through 14. But
  I recommend that you take a minute to familiarize yourself with the
  Pilates alphabet in Chapter 3 first. You also can find some Pilates tidbits
  that may be new to you in all of the other chapters.

How This Book Is Organized

This book is divided into five parts. In general, you can skip around and read different parts — but I recommend that you read Part I first and then Part II before looking too deeply into the other three parts.

Part I: Pilates Basics

If you're new to Pilates, I recommend that you read Part I first. It has the good stuff on how Pilates got started, how it's different from other exercise forms, what the benefits are, and lots of other tasty tidbits. Even if you're in a hurry to get to the exercises, I advise you to take a look at the Pilates alphabet in Chapter 3. The alphabet is a learning tool I've invented to make explaining basic Pilates movements easier. You can jump straight to the exercises without reading about the alphabet, but in the long run, you'll save yourself some time if you read about the alphabet first.

Part II: Mat Exercises

Part II is organized very simply: First, you start with the fundamental Pilates mat series, and then you move on systematically to the beginning series, then the intermediate series, and then the advanced series. I highly recommend not straying from this order because this is the order developed by the man himself, Joseph Pilates. There is a definite logic to the order, and if you start at the beginning, your body will be preparing to advance in a gradual and healthy way.

Don't just jump to the advanced exercises — at worst, you may hurt yourself, and at best, you won't be doing the exercises with proper form.

In Part II, I also give you some special exercises that may appeal to you, like special butt exercises from Chapter 9 or a lovely spine stretch from Chapter 10. In these chapters, the level of the exercise is noted so that you can make a decision as to whether you can handle it.

The chapter on super advanced exercises (Chapter 8) is another one that isn't really a series but is instead a selection of exercises you may insert into your advanced series (Chapter 7). This is where you can get a little creative, but I still recommend following the basic series listed in Chapters 4 through 7.

Part III: Beyond the Mat: Exercises Using Equipment and Accessories

Part III goes beyond the mat exercises to show you some photos and descriptions of Pilates equipment and accessories. Chapters 11, 12, and 13 show you exercises that you can do with affordable accessories. Chapter 14 shows you exercises that you do with your back to the wall, literally. And Chapter 15 is about the heavy equipment. This chapter is meant for those of you curious about going to a fully equipped Pilates studio or thinking about buying equipment for your home.

Part IV: Special Situations

Part IV may be the most important part of the book for you. If you're pregnant, or have been pregnant recently, read Chapter 16. It's all for you. Chapter 17 has special advice if you are older, have a bad back, or have stiff shoulders (like from sitting at a computer all day!).

Part V: The Part of Tens

The Part of Tens is in every *For Dummies* book. The chapters in this part each list ten Pilates-related factoids for your quick review.

Icons Used in This Book

When you see the Tip icon, you know that a piece of advice is coming that can make your life easier. It may be a way to modify an exercise, a way to make Pilates more affordable, or just something that can save you some time.

Some things are worth remembering. This icon flags the really crucial stuff that you should keep in mind.

Mainly, I use this icon to keep you from hurting yourself. If you see the Warning icon, make sure to read the adjacent paragraph carefully. You may be very glad you did!

Pilates is a mentally rigorous form of exercise. This icon flags images that you can hold in your mind's eye to help you perform an exercise correctly.

When you're ready to make an exercise harder, look for the Advanced Stuff icon. It flags modifications that you can make so that the exercises are more challenging.

Where to Go from Here

You can read this book by starting at the beginning and ending at the end. Or, if you want, flip around and browse through the parts that are most interesting — just don't try a Jackknife or Boomerang before you're ready! If you fit any of the special situations in Chapters 16 and 17, you may want to start there. Or, dive into the Part of Tens for easy-to-read nuggets of information about Pilates.

Part I
Pilates Basics

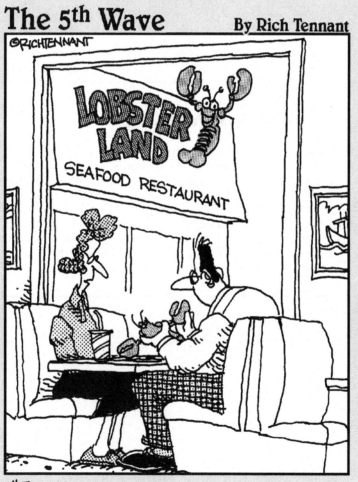

The 5th Wave   By Rich Tennant

"Is there a way you can explain
Pilates to me without using the
carcass of your lobster?"

In this part . . .

Part I gives you the information you need to know before getting serious about Pilates. Are you curious about what clothing or equipment you need before getting started? Do you want to know the practical benefits of doing Pilates? This part is for you. I also cover everything from the evolution of Pilates to the key concepts of Pilates to the Pilates alphabet, which is a learning tool I came up with that introduces you to the key movements that you perform again and again in the exercises.

Chapter 1

A Pilates Primer

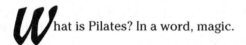hat is Pilates? In a word, magic.

But first things first. *Pilates* does not rhyme with *pirates*. It's puh-LAH-teez. If you were to look in on a busy Pilates studio, you might think, "Hey, this just looks like glorified sit-ups," or "What are these people doing, torturing them-selves with springs and pulleys?" or "Gee, this looks really fun and is just what I need!" And all these thoughts would be true.

Pilates is full of contradictions: It's strangely mundane and yet ethereal, simultaneously simple and complex. Some people understand and deeply appreciate the benefits of Pilates the first time they try it. Others may feel that Pilates exercises are repetitive and silly, but after three months of doing the same exercise, they suddenly gain access to a new layer of information about their bodies. Some people may initially find an exercise completely out of their reach, but after a few weeks of training, they find it to be completely natural. Whatever your experience of Pilates, the bottom line is always the same: You will be transformed.

My boyfriend, a serious freestyle snowboarder and skateboarder, informed me after his sixth session that "Pilates is boring." He prefers the thrill of danger and the reckless abandon that he finds on the slopes or on his skate-board. But he did grudgingly admit that his short brush with Pilates drasti-cally improved his snowboarding and allowed him to quit wearing his knee braces while snowboarding, after needing them for ten years.

His story is but one of the many testimonials I've received. A 35-year-old man who had back pain that nothing could help for 15 years, an elderly woman who had never enjoyed exercise and found herself losing flexibility and strength, and people who just wanted to tone up and have a gorgeous belly — all found what they needed in Pilates.

I myself am living proof of the Pilates magic. I seriously injured my knee 13 years ago during my short-lived career as a professional wrestler (a side job that I took when I was trying to support myself as a professional dancer). I was diagnosed as having a torn ligament, and the doctors recommended surgery if I wanted to continue dancing professionally. After six months of rehabilitation-based Pilates exercises and no surgery, I was up and dancing with more strength and technique than ever before. I was a convert.

I have had students come to Pilates without any prior movement experience. For some, it is the first form of exercise that appeals to them, either because they can't stand the gym scene — the loud music of aerobics, the grunting guys lifting weights — or they don't want to risk the potential injury or embarrassment that can come from not having any body knowledge. Pilates teaches fundamental movements; Pilates exercises are easy to learn and are completely safe for the average Joe.

If you already know a lot about Pilates or just want to get to the exercises, feel free to skip to Chapter 4, although I recommend that you check out the Pilates alphabet in Chapter 3 before attempting any of the exercises in this book.

As in starting any new exercise program, consult your doctor before starting Pilates, especially if you suffer from heart conditions, hypertension, or any other serious illness. If you have back pain or any other serious injury, please get a diagnosis from a doctor and your doctor's okay before embarking on your Pilates journey.

The Basics on Pilates

Pilates exercises borrow from yoga, dance, and gymnastics, but also include lots of original movements that distinguish them from these other techniques. The Pilates method consists of a repertoire of over 500 exercises to be done on a mat or on one of the many pieces of equipment Joseph Pilates invented. Don't worry about having to use complicated equipment — you can get a terrific workout at home with just a simple exercise mat. If you're interested in using special Pilates equipment, I give you the rundown in Chapter 15.

The Pilates method works to strengthen the center (see the section "Centering" in this chapter), lengthen the spine, build muscle tone, and increase body awareness and flexibility.

Joe Pilates: A short history of the man

Born in Germany in 1880 with a sunken chest and asthma, Joseph Hubertus Pilates spent his life obsessed with restoring his health and body condition. Over time, he overcame his frailty and became an accomplished skier, diver, gymnast, yogi, and boxer, maintaining top physical form well into his seventies. While in an English internment camp during World War I, Pilates rigged springs above hospital beds to allow patients to rehabilitate while lying on their backs. This setup later evolved into the cadillac, one of the main pieces of equipment in the Pilates method.

In 1923, Pilates emigrated to the United States. He settled in New York City, where he opened a studio on Eighth Avenue in Manhattan and started training and rehabilitating professional dancers. Ballet master George Balanchine and modern dance diva Martha Graham were two of his students.

Originally, Pilates developed a series of mat exercises designed to build abdominal strength and body control. He then built various pieces of equipment to enhance the results of his expanding repertoire of exercises. His motivation for building the equipment was to replace himself as a spotter for his clients. He developed 20-odd contraptions, some of which look a little like medieval torture devices. They were constructed of wood and metal piping, and used combinations of pulleys, straps, bars, boxes, and springs. His philosophy led him to develop a regimen that "develops the body uniformly, corrects wrong postures, restores physical vitality, invigorates the mind, and elevates the spirit." Way ahead of his time, he viewed fitness holistically, emphasizing the body working as a whole unit.

Over the decades, Pilates developed over 500 exercises, which he originally called Contrology but which have since come to be known as the Pilates method.

The Pilates method is also an excellent rehabilitation system for back, knee, hip, shoulder, and repetitive-stress injuries. Pilates addresses the body as a whole, correcting the body's asymmetries and chronic weaknesses to prevent reinjury and to bring the body back into balance.

Pilates mat work uses series of exercises

Pilates mat exercises are usually done in a series. Series are organized by levels. This book contains pre-Pilates, beginning, intermediate, and advanced series.

I recommend starting with pre-Pilates (Chapter 4). The pre-Pilates exercises give you a deep understanding of the concepts that make up all Pilates exercises. After you understand these concepts, you can apply them to the beginning series. After you have mastered the beginning series, move on to the intermediate series, and so on. As you progress in the method, the series get longer and harder. An intermediate workout includes exercises from the beginning series, plus new and harder intermediate exercises. Sometimes you will just do a more difficult version of the same exercise when you advance in levels.

Going through a series in order and trying to complete the whole series when you work out is important. Joseph Pilates was a genius when it comes to understanding muscle balance in the body. The series he developed make sense to the body when the exercises are done in the correct order. Usually, you start a series with an exercise that warms up the spine, then you do a few exercises that bend the spine in one direction, followed by an exercise that reverses that movement, and so on. You don't have to understand the science behind why these exercises are in the order that they're in (you would need a Ph.D. in kinesiology to fully understand the reasons). Just trust in the method and in the order of the exercises. The longer I study and practice Pilates, the more I appreciate the intelligence of the man who created it.

Pilates builds the powerhouse

Pilates exercises, as a whole, develop strong abdominal, back, butt, and deep-postural muscles. Pilates focuses on the muscles that support the skeletal system and act as the powerhouse of the body.

Powerhouse is a term that comes from Joe Pilates himself. (See the sidebar "Joe Pilates: A short history of the man" in this chapter for information about the man who developed Pilates exercises.) The abdominals, butt, back, and sometimes the inner thigh muscles, when working together, constitute the powerhouse. This is where many of the Pilates exercises can be initiated or the area that is being challenged in many exercises. These muscles are the main stabilizing muscles of the torso and are very important for preventing injury to the back.

Why should you care about your powerhouse?

- The powerhouse muscles protect your back from potential injury, and if you already have a weak or problematic back, then strengthening the powerhouse will probably alleviate your problems.

- Working from the center of the body when doing any movement takes the load off of the joints and the spine and helps your body work more efficiently.

- A strong powerhouse is a sexy thing. Who doesn't enjoy a toned belly, butt, back, and inner thigh?

The Evolution of Pilates

The original Eighth Avenue Pilates studio is where the first generation of teachers were trained: Romana Kyranowska, Kathy Grant, Ron Fletcher, Eve Gentry, Carola Trier, Mary Bowen, and Bruce King. Pilates' protégés soon branched out and opened studios around the country, changing the method based on their own individual backgrounds and philosophies, and sometimes on the needs of their clients. For the following fifty years or so, the Pilates method has been passed down through generations of teachers and has transformed a great deal along the way. New York teachers claim to hold truest to the original Pilates method, but many creative individuals have brought their insights about the body to improve upon some of the views of posture that were built into the original Pilates method and that now seem antiquated.

My approach to the Pilates method is a combination of New York and California styles. I was originally trained in New York by Romana, who holds the closest to Joe's original method. There I learned the more classic repertoire of exercises and the traditional New York posture cues. New York Pilates tends to focus on flattening the low back, tucking the pelvis, and using the butt muscles a whole lot in the work. California and West Coast Pilates teachers, in contrast, talk a lot about Neutral Spine or neutral pelvis, which is more the way a person naturally stands — with a curve in the low back, not a flattened low back (see Chapter 3 for a detailed description of Neutral Spine).

Out here in California, we like to be free and open to new ideas. Over the years, I and many of the teachers who work in my studio have developed new exercises based on Pilates concepts, or have modified old exercises to make them more effective and to apply what we now know about the body. Basically, flattening your back and tucking your pelvis under all the time is not great for most people and may exacerbate back problems.

The Eight Great Principles of Pilates

Joseph Pilates wrote a book called *Return to Life* in which he mapped out the eight principles that inspired the Pilates method. Understanding these principles helps you gain a deeper understanding of the philosophy underlying Pilates. Pilates, more than other exercise programs, requires *mental* focus. If you don't understand the concepts behind Pilates, it ends up being merely a series of fancy sit-ups and stretches.

What's in a name?

In 1992, a physical therapist from New York named Sean Gallagher acquired the trademark for the Pilates studio and exercise instruction services. Shortly thereafter, he began taking legal action against Pilates instructors, suing everyone he could find who was using the Pilates name and claiming that he alone had the right to use *Pilates.* Many Pilates trainers and studio owners settled out of court or paid this man a fee for use of the Pilates name. Others merely changed the name of what they were doing to things like *Cor Fitness, the Method,* or *PhysicalMind.* In 1996, Gallagher met his match when he sued Balanced Body, the world's largest manufacturer of Pilates equipment. Balanced Body's owner, Ken Edelman, found it ludicrous that longtime teachers of Pilates could no longer use the name. He countersued. After four years of litigation and an 11-day trial, a U.S. District Court ruled that *Pilates* is the name of a method of exercise and that the name cannot be owned by Gallagher or anyone else.

What drives people to continue doing Pilates for years and years is the tremendous transformation they see in their bodies when they delve deeper into the work. You could do Pilates for ten years and still find some revelation about your body or about how to deepen the effects of an exercise. This aspect distinguishes Pilates from other exercise forms.

When you do Pilates exercises with the eight key concepts in mind, you gain many more levels of meaning and effectiveness. The following eight concepts give you an idea of just what to think about when doing the exercises.

Control

Joseph Pilates originally called his method *Controlology* (it wasn't until his students took over teaching for him that people started referring to the method as *Pilates*). So one of the most fundamental rules when doing Pilates is to control your body's every movement. This rule applies not only to the exercises themselves but also to transitions between exercises, how you get on and off the equipment, and your overall attention to detail while working out.

When doing mat exercises, control comes into play with the initiation and ending of each movement. When you put on the brakes in a controlled manner, you train the muscles to hold in a lengthened state. Over time, the muscles grow long as well as strong. Long and strong muscles — isn't that what we all want? When training clients, I try to encourage smooth and even movements. In my mind, I think of getting the muscles to cooperate with each other.

Also, when focusing on control of a movement, the body is forced to recruit helper muscles (called *synergists*), which are usually smaller than the main muscles. When many muscles work together to do one movement, or when muscles work synergistically, the body as a whole develops greater balance and coordination. Also, the big muscles won't get too big and bulky because they don't have to do all the work by themselves. Thus you become a long and lean machine. Once your body learns to move with control, you'll feel more confident doing all kinds of things, from climbing a ladder to swing dancing to diving off a cliff.

Inner control allows you outer freedom without fear of injury.

Breath

People often hold their breath when performing a new and difficult task. When you hold your breath, you tense muscles that can ultimately exacerbate improper posture and reinforce tension habits. That is why consistent breathing is essential to flowing movement and proper muscle balance. Every Pilates exercise has a specific breathing pattern assigned to it.

Most people breathe at half of their lung capacity. Shallow breathing is an unfortunate side effect of a sedentary and stressful life. Deep inhalation and full exhalation exercises the lungs and increases lung capacity, bringing deep relaxation as a pleasant side effect. Breathing while moving is not always an easy assignment; but when you do it, beautiful things can happen. Focused breath can help maximize the body's ability to stretch, and through this release of tension, you'll gain optimal body control.

Breathing is an essential aspect of Pilates and distinguishes it from other exercise forms. Like yoga, Pilates has specific breathing cues to go with every exercise.

My general rule of Pilates breathing: Exhale on the work!

Kathy Grant, a first-generation Pilates master, has developed three catagories of Pilates breathing (for more on Kathy Grant, see the sidebar in Chapter 21):

✔ **Accordion breathing:** Put your hands on either side of your rib cage, as if holding on to an accordion. Take a deep breath in, expanding the space between your hands. Imagine expanding the rib cage sideways. On the exhale, feel the rib cage decrease in size, squeezing your accordion together. This is a way to breathe laterally into your ribs and maintain stability in the front, instead of lifting and dropping the rib cage, which can destabilize the torso.

✔ **Percussive breathing:** This breathing is exemplified in the Hundred exercise that recurs in Chapters 5, 6, and 7. The inhale can be like an accordion — smooth and deep — while the exhale should be percussive. You can even make a shh sound on every beat to increase the percussive quality. You should be able to feel the abdominals forcing the air out of your lungs, called *forced expiration.*

✔ **Hide-and-seek breathing:** What would your breathing be like if you were hiding underneath a sheet and someone came looking for you? This is hide-and-seek breathing. It is essential to maintain breath control in Pilates or any other high-performance sport where balance and stability are paramount. If you were a gymnast about to do a back flip on a balance beam, you wouldn't want your breathing to displace any part of your body. Basically, it is possible to inhale and exhale without a whole lot of movement in the rib cage or the belly.

Flowing movement

If you were to glance quickly at someone doing Pilates, you might think the person was doing yoga. But when doing yoga, you generally hold your position for at least a moment (if not for what seems like an eternity) before moving to the next posture. And although Pilates borrows some of its movements from yoga, rarely do you hold a position for a long time in Pilates. In this way, Pilates is more like dance, in that the flow of the body is essential. The essence of Pilates movements is to allow your body to move freely and, at the end of each movement, to finish with control and precision. This way of moving brings flexibility to the joints and muscles and teaches the body to elongate and move with even rhythm. Flowing movement integrates the nervous system, the muscles, and the joints and trains the body to move smoothly and evenly.

Precision

Precision is a lot like control but has the added element of spatial awareness. When initiating any movement, you must know exactly where that movement starts and where it will end. All Pilates exercises have precise definitions of where the body should be at all times. The little things count in Pilates.

Many people develop exercise habits that contribute to injury or painful conditions. For instance, some people constantly tighten their shoulders when performing any difficult or challenging exercise. Engaging your upper trapezius (those muscles at the top of your shoulder which run up the back of the neck that most people are constantly rubbing) certainly won't help you do a leg exercise, but you'd be surprised how many people try to use them! This is a bad habit that any good Pilates trainer will correct.

A goal of Pilates is to focus on the specific muscles that should be working and relaxing all the muscles that may want to help out but shouldn't. It all comes back to being fully present when working out and being specific about what muscles you use and what muscles you don't use. The whole body must be in agreement when moving the Pilates way. This kind of precision in movement will resonate in the rest of your life. For example, suppose that you suffer from pain because of faulty postural habits that you aren't even aware of. After a few good sessions of Pilates, you may be pleasantly surprised by how fast a newfound awareness can effect positive change in the body. This change can happen only when you begin to notice yourself in your body and increase the precision in your movements.

Centering

Again and again, I need to remind my clients to "pull the navel to the spine" — in other words, suck in that gut! This is the first and ultimate Pilates cue. Pulling the navel in toward your spine is how you bring your deep abdominal muscles into action, and all Pilates exercises are done with the deep abdominals engaged to ensure proper centering. Most Pilates exercises focus on developing abdominal strength either directly or indirectly. Never forget to pull the belly in, or you'll be reprimanded by the Pilates gods!

Even when you're performing an exercise that focuses on strengthening the arm muscles, the instructor will ask you to pull your navel in, keep your shoulders pulling down the back, and perhaps even squeeze your butt. All these actions promote centering and core muscle strength. No exercise should be done to the detriment of center control. In other words, if the center is not totally and completely engaged and stabilized, you may not progress to the next level of an exercise. Furthermore, until absolute centering can be maintained, you must modify an exercise so it can be done with this essential concept in mind. Sound tough? They don't call me the abdominatrix for nothing.

Stability

The focus on stability when performing the exercises is part of the beauty of Pilates and what makes it such a perfect rehabilitation system. In fact, many Pilates mat exercises are meant to focus primarily on torso stability. *Stability* is the ability to *not* move a part of the body while another part is challenging it. For instance, when raising your arm up as high as you can in front of you, try not to arch your back. In order to accomplish this, you must use your abdominal muscles so that the rib cage doesn't rise up as the arm rises above the shoulder level. Maintaining stillness in the spine as you move the arms and legs requires torso stability that is accomplished mainly by the abdominal muscles.

The lion's share of Pilates exercises utilize this concept of torso stability, which is one of the keys to the health and longevity of your spine. After an injury, there is generally instability in the injured area. The first thing you want to do is learn to stabilize the injured part so as not to reinjure and to allow the healing process to begin. Thus, Pilates is one of the safest forms of exercise to do after an injury. Also, Pilates will prevent injury because you're much less likely to injure yourself in the first place if you have excellent stability in your torso and joints.

If you've ever been to the circus or an advanced yoga, dance, or stretch class, you've probably seen a superflexible person. You know the kind of person I'm talking about — someone who seems to have no bones in her body, a contortionist type who can put her feet behind her ears and bend backward like a wishbone. These people have extreme flexibility, which is the opposite of stability. Too much flexibility puts excessive wear and tear on ligaments and joints. Thus, extremely flexible people tend to injure themselves regularly. Learning to stabilize the various parts of the body is essential for injury prevention and rehabilitation from injury. Torso stability is accomplished mainly by abdominal strength and is one of the most important concepts in the Pilates method. The main concept to think of when attempting to achieve stability is simply "don't move it."

The torso can be broken down into two parts: upper torso (ribcage/upper back) and lower torso (low belly/low back).

✔ **Upper torso stability uses upper abdominals.** Upper torso stability is challenged by the upper limbs (arms). When lying flat on your back, if you reach your arms above your head, in order to keep your upper back and rib cage from rising up, you must engage and use your upper abdominals to maintain torso stability. The concept of upper torso stability is used anytime the arms are moving while the torso must remain stable.

✔ **Lower torso stability uses lower abdominals.** Lower torso stability is challenged by the lower limbs (legs). When lying flat on your back with legs straight up in the air, as you lower your legs away from you, you need to use your lower abdominals to keep your low back from hyperextending or arching off the mat.

Full torso stability, then, uses the whole abdominal wall. Full torso stability is challenged by movement of the arms and legs at the same time. If you are lying flat on your back with your arms and legs pointing straight up, as you move your arms and legs away from each other, the whole abdominal wall must engage and work to keep the whole torso from arching off the mat. This concept is used in several intermediate and advanced Pilates exercises.

Range of motion

Range of motion is a medical term that refers to how much movement a part of the body can do. For instance, how high you can kick your leg out in front of you gives you an idea of how much range of motion you have in your hip. Range of motion can be affected by the muscles, bones, and other tissues such as ligaments and fascia (connective tissue). Basically, range of motion is just another way of describing flexibility.

Pilates exercises tend to require the body to move to its fullest length, thereby increasing the range of motion, or flexibility, of your limbs. People whose muscles are very tight will begin to notice an increase in flexibility after doing a few hours of Pilates exercises. If you're very tight, you may need to do some specific stretching exercises in addition to the Pilates exercises. You may find yourself limited by your tightness and unable even to get into the position required to perform a particular exercise. If you find this to be true, you may need to modify the exercise at first, until you gain the flexibility to do the exercise in its classic form.

Opposition

You can lift your arms thinking only of lifting your arms. Or you can think "down to go up" as you lift your arms, first pulling the shoulders down the back and then raising the arms, focusing on lifting the arms from the back muscles instead. This is opposition in action. When lifting your arm from your back rather than from your arm, you're actually stabilizing the shoulder as you lift the arm. I often say to my clients, "Think down to go up" when they're raising their arms, or "up to go down" when I'm explaining how to roll down the spine. These are both examples of opposition when moving.

Dancers naturally use opposition when they move, and that is what gives them the illusion of floating in the air while simultaneously being weighted to the ground. Opposition imagery in moving is generally a way to trick someone into using core muscles rather than the peripheral muscles. This approach brings in more muscles to do a movement and makes the movement more efficient for the body, and ultimately more healthy.

As a Pilates instructor, I use opposition often and in many ways to get clients to find a balance in their bodies. The other example of "up to go down" when bending over is essential to save your back from eventual demise. The next time you bend down to pick something up, imagine pulling up from your low belly as you bend forward. Doing so will protect your back by engaging the opposing muscles (the abdominals). Using opposition is a beautiful way to manipulate your body as you perform movements with ultimate elongation and proper body mechanics. You'll see more examples of opposition when you go through the exercises, and the concept will be easier to understand after you've done a few.

What You Need to Get Started

The good news is that you don't need much! Just the basics:

- **A firm mat.** The mat only needs to be as long as your spine and as wide as your body. This mat should be firm enough to support your back when rolling on the floor. You will hurt your vertebrae if you use only a towel or a yoga mat. I like to use either a gymnastic mat or a fold up foam mat.

- **Comfy clothes.** Wear what you would wear to a yoga class, dance class, or stretch class. Nothing should bind you — no buttons or tight waist-bands. Wearing something formfitting is nice because it lets you see if your belly is pooching out or not.

- **Bare feet.** Socks tend to slip on the floor, so I recommend bare feet.

In addition, a small ball is great, although it's not necessary. A small ball is a great cheap tool to have, especially when you're first starting out. See Chapter 12 for more information.

Great places to buy Pilates stuff

You may be able to find another source that you trust, but I can vouch for these three suppliers:

- **Balanced Body, Inc.** (1-800-Pilates, www. pilates.com) In my opinion, Balanced Body is the best place to order large Pilates equipment and small Pilates accessories. It also has an international directory of Pilates instructors. The new catalogue will be offering the Pilates spring board, a piece of equipment which was developed by yours truly.

- **OPTP** (1-800-367-7393, www.optp.com)

- **Fitness Wholesale** (1-888-FWORDER, www.fwonline.com)

Chapter 2

Get Ready, Get Set . . .

In This Chapter
▶ Finding out how Pilates can affect your daily life
▶ Discovering how your body can change

*I*f you want to skip ahead and go straight to the exercises, that's okay. But you may want to read this chapter first. Imagine that you're at the starting line, ready to go. This chapter tells you what you need to know before the starter pistol goes off — before you get serious about adding Pilates to your life.

Combining Pilates with Other Forms of Exercise

Pilates teaches you essential things about your body that everyone should know. If you are an athlete, you will especially benefit from the knowledge Pilates has to offer. Joseph Pilates himself was a gymnast and boxer, and enjoyed many outdoor sports as well. Originally he worked with rehabilitating professional dancers in New York, but his expertise soon spread to athletes of all kinds.

At my studio in San Francisco, we work with all kinds of sports fanatics, and all rave about the improvements they see after just a few Pilates sessions. Swimmers, skiers, snowboarders, cyclists, runners, weight lifters, divers, gymnasts, and ice skaters all come to the studio to gain core strength and flexibility. Pilates is strength training *and* conditioning. It tones the muscles and teaches the muscles how to work together for greater efficiency of movement. Pilates teaches proper alignment, improves balance and coordination, and therefore helps prevent injury.

I usually tell my clients to combine Pilates with some form of aerobic exercise for a complete workout program. If you are already doing an aerobic sport that you love, then Pilates will just enhance your program. No matter what sport you do, Pilates will improve your overall muscle tone, increase your flexibility, and improve your technique. Basically, Pilates is a great complement to any sport.

Keeping Your Eyes on the Prize: How You Benefit from Pilates

Yeah, yeah, I've heard it a hundred times. When you try and make Pilates a part of your routine, you find that you just don't have time . . . or you don't have the energy . . . or it's too much work! Well, the time for excuses is over. Just in case you need more motivation, this section shows you the rewards you can reap from Pilates — if you keep your eyes on the prize.

Finding your center

Most people at some time in their lives experience back pain, and the most common reasons for back pain are poor posture and weak tummy muscles.

The very first thing you figure out as a Pilates student is how to suck in your gut. In nicer words, that means how to pull your navel in toward the spine. By performing this simple action, you engage your deep abdominal muscles. Strengthening these muscles can transform your posture and alleviate back pain. All Pilates exercises are done with this basic centering concept.

An hour-long Pilates mat class, if taught by a competent teacher, fires up those abdominal muscles and makes you want to scream "uncle!" As you become more advanced in the Pilates method, your core strength develops a great deal more. You may notice a greater ease in your body and will probably find increased endurance for lifting, walking, and performing daily activities. Your posture improves, and people will see a change in your physicality. Your back pain may just up and go away, as well as other bodily aches and pains like knee, shoulder, and hip problems. Developing core strength affects your whole being and gives you a new sense of power.

Once you've studied Pilates, it is impossible not to apply the concepts of core strength and deep abdominal engagement to the rest of your life. Many students tell me that they hear my voice as they drive in their car or sit at work, telling them "sit up tall, pull your shoulders down the back, lift from your center, pull your navel in." That they hear my voice at all hours of the day and night could not make me happier! I have had a positive effect, one that is lasting and gloriously healthy for their spine and the longevity of their being.

Mastering the mental component

REMEMBER

Don't do Pilates if you don't want to think. Pilates is not a mindless, repetitive workout. When doing Pilates exercises, it's not what you do, but how you do it. The emphasis is on your form, so you need a certain presence of mind.

I call Pilates "high exercise" because it teaches you how to be *in* your body: how to properly sit and stand, how to bend and lift, and how to move from the center of the body. This increased body awareness and core strength help to improve form in other sports as well and to bring more grace and efficiency to everyday life activities.

People who bring focus and mental presence to their workouts advance more quickly through the exercises and see improvements more readily. Like dance, Pilates demands that your body perform many actions at once. A movement is never just a movement; you must execute it with optimal form, precision, and control. Each person has the potential to reach his or her own level of perfection. Achieving this goal requires focus and attention, and it can be frustrating for those who don't want to be so present in their body.

Helping your spine, the axis of life

The spine has two main functions: first, to be rigid and hold you upright and strong against the elements, and second, to be flexible and allow you to bend over, twist around, and reach in many directions. Most of the time, the spine does a heck of a good job. The spine is very susceptible to injury because it moves so much and in so many different ways. The risk of injury increases as you get older and the shock-absorbing structures begin to deteriorate. The spine also gets much stiffer as you age, making it more difficult to move about the way you want. Pilates is one of the best methods of exercise to address both spinal stability and spinal rigidity.

A Pilates exercise usually serves one purpose at a time. One exercise may aim at increasing flexibility in the spine, while another may focus on developing core stabilization and strength. A balanced workout addresses both concerns, giving the spine more resilience. Joe Pilates loved to use the cat as a model for spinal strength and mobility (see Chapter 10 for some exercises that are inspired by the cat). He used to say if you do Pilates for 20 minutes a day, your spine will be like a cat's, and you will be able to move freely through your life. Meow!

Becoming an upright citizen: The psychological issues of standing tall

One of my first regular Pilates clients, Solomon, a cab driver from San Francisco, came to me to improve his posture and general sense of well-being. Not long into our professional relationship, Solomon (Solly for short) began telling me of his present woes and past dysfunctional relationships, his struggle with drug and alcohol abuse, and his ultimate triumph over substances. (My most enjoyable Pilates sessions are spent not as a personal trainer, but as a lay psychotherapist.) Solly had chosen Pilates as part of his healing process. He was a devoted client, a hard worker, and a fast learner. After our sessions, he seemed taller, more open, and self-assured. He would always thank me, reschedule, and get dressed, putting on his baggy jeans, T-shirt, windbreaker, and baseball cap placed backward on his head. One day, I noticed with dread that my client was slouching. As the cap reached his head, an instantaneous transformation took place: shoulders rounded forward, head dropped, his peripheral vision restricted to the lower portion of the universe. I cringed as he left, slumping off down the hall. That's when it hit me: Some people are not ready to face the world as an upright citizen.

Why? Well, it takes a lifetime to develop poor posture, and by age 50, most people's spines reflect the way they've lived their life — or faced up to it. Most people, in other words, have the spine they deserve. We all tend to unconsciously sculpt our bodies to fit our personalities.

What are you? A too-tall-too-early slumper? Or maybe a hide-my-large-breasts-with-rolled-in-shoulders woman? Or perhaps you prefer the swaybacked, belly-protruding vulnerable child look? Or maybe a tight-butted, tucked-pelvis, lock-kneed, control-freak variety? These are all ways we live in our bodies and communicate our feelings about ourselves to others.

But emotional baggage isn't the only thing that thwarts good posture: We shrink as we age because gravity is working against us every minute. The only way to combat shrinkage is to stand up to it, literally. Small muscles in between the vertebrae keep the spine lengthened, and these are the ones that get contracted and weak with poor posture and laziness. You need to tone these muscles in the same way as you do with your thighs or your arms — through repeated use against a form of resistance, and in this case, the resistance is not a free weight (or a spring, as in Pilates) but gravity itself.

When working with a client's posture, usually the simplest instructions are the most effective. "Imagine there is a golden string attached to the back of the top of your head and it's pulling you gently up toward the sky. . . ." In other words, stand up straight, and hold your gut in.

I attended a symposium on the subject of geriatrics and heard an excellent speaker postulating that the stereotypical hunching, arthritic postures of old age are just that — not necessary outcomes of living a long life, but a fulfillment of our preconceptions of aging. The lecturer claims that wrinkling and sagging are all a process of what he calls habituation, which basically means doing the same old thing day after day with your same old body.

You see, simply standing up on earth is a lot of work for certain muscles, called postural muscles, which consist of the following:

✔ The deep muscles of the back that hold up the spine

✔ The upper trapezius, which holds up the shoulders

✔ The jaw muscles that keep the lower jaw from dropping

✔ The tight iliotibial bands on the sides of your legs

✔ The quadriceps, the hamstrings, and the psoas that keep your legs standing

These postural muscles have great endurance and can withstand hours of work keeping us standing and sitting upright against gravity. You may have wondered why your jaw gets sore or why the back of your neck gets tight. These types of pain are natural manifestations of postural muscles doing their duty. These muscles tend toward over-tightness because they are constantly firing to keep our bones upright.

With correct posture, these postural muscles function beautifully to keep us standing and sitting up pain-free. But the problem arises when we live our sedentary lives; Janda, a great Czechoslovakian rehabilitation specialist calls humans "homo sedentaris." He postulates that sitting for hours a day with poor posture creates an imbalance in the body. As a result, the postural muscles stop working, and the other muscles which are not equipped to withstand hours of constant work are forced to help out with staying upright. These muscles will become very sore after a few hours of this overwork, and hence back pain. You can't ask a sprinter to run a marathon, right? This is what we do when we sit slouching at our desks all day. And then we wonder why we have back pain!

Pilates teaches us how to stand properly, sit properly, lift, bend over, get up, and perform daily activities or high-level sports without hurting ourselves. Pilates teaches us how to properly use our postural muscles.

Are you ready to have good posture? Are you emotionally prepared to receive what the world may offer you when standing upright with your head up? Or will you be another Solly, giving in to old, familiar, and somehow comforting habits? Try this exercise, right now while you're reading this: Sit up straight, with your head balanced on top of your hips, your shoulders open and dropped away from your ears, and your eyes looking straight ahead to ensure proper neck alignment. And lastly, imagine that you're listening to angels above and behind you.

Improving your sex life

Pilates can help your sex life. Increasing body awareness and discovering how to isolate muscles in your pelvic floor can only increase your pleasure and give you more control during sex. (Your pelvic floor muscles include the muscles that control the sphincters of your urethra, anus, and the muscles of the vagina.) And of course, gaining flexibility in the hips and legs and increasing strength in your pelvis and butt will give you more choices on what positions you can attempt, and more physical endurance for longer rounds! It will also prevent pulled muscles and injuries if you enjoy more athletic sexual experiences.

Looking good: Pilates and the body beautiful

You may have heard of all the Hollywood stars who are doing Pilates: Madonna, Patrick Swayze, Robin Williams, Sharon Stone, that woman who plays Xena, and many more. Bette Midler even had a cadillac (see Chapter 15 for more on this piece of Pilates equipment) on her short-lived TV show. You know that if those stars are doing Pilates, it must be doing something good for their vanity! Read on to find out the specifics.

Pilates and weight loss

Many people come to Pilates to lose weight and have a body like a dancer's. Is this realistic? Yes and no.

Aerobic exercise facilitates fat loss, and Pilates is not aerobic until you get to the advanced levels and are able to transition seamlessly from one exercise to another. If you do no exercise at all now, you may lose fat doing Pilates . . . because hey, it is exercise and it will increase your metabolism. But if fat loss is a primary concern to you, try combining Pilates with dancing, walking, swimming, biking, or using some gym-based aerobic machine. See Chapter 22 for more ideas.

Pilates is resistance training, so it strengthens and tones your whole body. You will see marked changes especially around the belly, butt, and thighs. Most important, Pilates can make you appear taller and more elegant by giving you beautiful posture, grace, and ease of movement.

A long and lean Pilates machine

How can you get a hottie Pilates body? How does Pilates make you appear longer and leaner? The secret is in the way you move your body in Pilates, which contributes to length and sinew and overall grace. The important thing is just to know that Pilates does not make you bulky — it gives you a healthy muscle tone. For details, see the sidebar "Why Pilates makes you long and lean."

The Pilates way of moving

"Reach your fingertips long and away!" "Stretch your leg out to its fullest length!" These are common commands of a good Pilates trainer. You should always be accentuating the extension of the limbs and challenging your body to gain more and more length. This way of moving lengthens the muscles and opens the joints, training your body as dancers train theirs. When you practice elongating the muscles, your muscles remember to stay long and open after you leave the Pilates studio. You can increase flexibility and literally become a longer human being.

The Pilates triad: Abs, butt, and inner thigh

What makes Pilates different from a lot of other exercise forms is that you're always using every part of your body. Even if you're just doing a bicep curl, you don't let the rest of your body go to jelly; you're holding your gut in, squeezing your butt, and pulling your inner thighs together at the same time. When doing Pilates exercises, you almost always work on the triad of abs, butt, and inner thigh, no matter what else is going on. Over time, this combination of muscle usage changes the look and shape of your middle.

Don't dingle dangle! Pilates and the upper body

Joseph Pilates was a gymnast, and many of the intermediate and advanced exercises reflect this fact. Many Pilates exercises demand a great amount of upper body strength and stability, much like a gymnastics routine. This focus on strengthening the back and upper body sets Pilates apart from most forms of exercise. Most people (especially women) have little upper-body strength. When women start Pilates, they are pleasantly surprised by the tone and definition they gain in their arms and back as they progress in the work. See Figure 2-1 for an example of a Pilates-toned upper body.

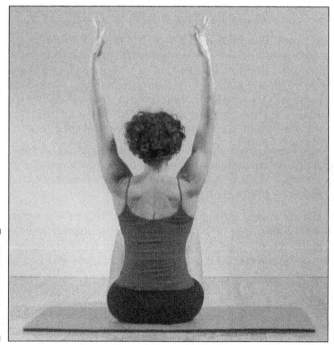

Figure 2-1:
Pilates strengthens and tones the upper body.

Seeing Is Believing: Some Pilates Images

Pilates isn't like, say, jogging. Many people find jogging relaxing because they can let their mind wander. The body goes on autopilot, and the mind is free to do other things. Not so with Pilates. Pilates — although relaxing in its own way — requires concentration. You have to think about what you're doing.

Visual images play an important role in Pilates because they help your body assume the correct position. Keep the following images in mind as you do your Pilates exercises.

- ✔ **Pull the navel toward the spine.** This image reminds people to engage their deep abdominal muscles. This image is the most essential one in Pilates.

- ✔ **A golden string at the back of the top of your head pulls you up to the sky.** This image helps people lengthen their whole spine when sitting or standing. Sitting up straight and standing with your head aligned with your hips are essential to strengthening the deep muscles of the back. These postural muscles tend to get very weak and over-stretched in people who slouch or sit all day at a computer. This weakness is one of the main causes of back pain.

- ✔ **Keep the shoulders back and down.** This image counteracts the tendency to let the shoulders creep up by the ears when doing exercises, especially difficult ones. People tend to use their upper traps (trapezius) to help perform an exercise for no good reason; it is a tension response that is unnecessary and important to address. By keeping the shoulders back and down, you are engaging your back muscles, which stabilizes the shoulders and helps counteract the overworking upper traps.

- ✔ **Keep your ears growing away from your shoulders and the shoulders dropping down away from the ears.** This is another image to help relax the upper traps. This image helps remind people to keep their spine long, especially the neck.

- ✔ **Lower the rib cage.** Letting your rib cage protrude from your chest when using your upper body is a common response. Remember, however, that keeping the rib cage down or "knitted" into the abdomen helps to maintain upper torso stability and keeps the upper abdominal muscles engaged.

Why Pilates makes you long and lean

Here are some elements of Pilates and why they give you the long and lean body that many people come to Pilates for.

The scoop

You don't get six-pack abs by doing Pilates. In the mat work, the first thing you figure out how to do is to pull the navel in toward the spine. In other words, you compress your abdominal wall, which eventually creates the look of a flatter belly. Pulling inward trains your middle to be not only strong and supportive of your back but look like a sleek and toned tummy without the protruding six-pack, which is the sign of superficially strong abdominal muscles.

The springs

All Pilates equipment involves exercising against a spring resistance. A spring is different than a free weight. The amount of resistance of a spring changes as you stretch it out, challenging the muscle along an increasing continuum. Training against spring resistance builds long and gorgeous muscles that have flexibility and coordination to boot!

Complex movements

Pilates exercises require many muscles to work at the same time. You rarely do a simple movement like straightening and bending the arm over and over. A Pilates exercise might combine a stretch of the spine with an arm circle followed by a sit-up. You're challenging your body in many different ways. Pilates requires the body to perform different tasks that recruit many muscle groups at once. This kind of complex movement develops small and large muscles simultaneously. No one muscle gets all the attention; the smaller muscles become stronger, and the bigger ones can take a break and not get too big and bulky.

Variation

You never do more than ten repetitions of any exercise in Pilates, and you never repeat the same exercise in a session. Instead, you move from one exercise to the next in well-thought-out order. You go from an abdominal exercise to a back exercise to an upper body exercise, and on and on. Meanwhile, no exercise is just working one muscle. Even if it's called a tricep press, you are always working from the core and recruiting muscles to perform what looks like a simple arm movement. To build and bulk up a muscle (in body building, for example), you need to fatigue that one muscle and do repetitions with resting in between. This approach is completely antithetical to the Pilates approach of body conditioning. Pilates is like a dance that flows, and your whole body is required to participate. See the photos in Chapter 8 for some good examples of the way that Pilates flows.

Chapter 3

Getting on a Mat and Learning the Pilates Alphabet

In This Chapter

▶ Finding out about mat exercises

▶ Discovering the elements of the Pilates alphabet

The mat is the essence of Pilates. A daily mat regimen guarantees you a strong center and enables you to progress as a Pilates student, whether you continue with the mat work only or decide to try one of the many pieces of Pilates equipment.

Mat work strengthens your deep abdominal, butt, and back muscles; teaches torso stability; increases your overall flexibility; and improves your posture. Mat work, when done at an advanced level, is a full-body workout, and a quite challenging one at that.

Although it's best to have a firm mat under you, Pilates mat work can be done anywhere you have a soft but supportive surface under your spine. You have no excuse not to do a little mat work every day.

Most mat work focuses on core strength (that is, strength in your belly, back, and butt), so it trains your middle to be more compressed. You may see definition you never had before in your abdominals, and the whole middle region will begin to tone in a very delightful way. Because Pilates focuses on the deep abdominals, the sides of your torso will become more defined and the superficial pooching muscles of your belly will disappear.

Women naturally have abdominal fat, which may or may not diminish. Losing abdominal fat is a function of weight loss — not muscular definition — but Pilates can be an important part of your weight-loss plan when it's combined with aerobic exercise.

Deciding Whether Mat Exercises Are Right for You

Some people aren't able to use the Pilates mat. For example, I have a 63-year-old female client who has a very difficult time doing an Upper Abdominal Curl (which you are introduced to in Chapter 4) and definitely can't do the Hundred (one of the most basic mat exercises). These two exercises, although considered beginning Pilates, require you to lift your head and roll into a curled position (what I call the Pilates Abdominal Position). This movement is impossible for my client. An untrained eye may think that she's just too weak in her tummy. But upon closer observation, it becomes evident that she is unable to roll up and hold the Pilates Abdominal Position because she is very tight in her upper back and neck.

Other than tightness, factors that may limit a person's ability to do Pilates mat work include a weak tummy or extreme tightness in any part of the spine or hips. If these conditions sound familiar, don't give up on Pilates. These types of difficulties are actually fairly common. What can you do about them? Well, if you're exceptionally tight and find mat work impossible, you can head down to your local Pilates studio. Much of the Pilates equipment is designed to help beginners. But I'm betting that you don't have easy access to a Pilates studio and the wonderful equipment (all of which I describe in Chapter 15) therein.

So if you're attempting your Pilates fundamentals on your own at home and find that some exercise just baffles your mind or your body, just move on to the next one. Don't get flustered, don't get mad, just move. Trust that in time you'll be able to do whatever is out of reach for you right now. You may be limited by tight muscles and joints. You may be limited by weakness (a very common problem). You may be limited by lack of concentration and lack of coordination. Don't worry. That's why you're reading this book. Pilates will help you with all these things if you just trust in the method.

Pilates exercises address tightness by stretching the body in each exercise. Pilates exercises address weakness by strengthening the body in each exercise. The most important thing to remember is to just do the work regularly. Your body will change in time. As you advance in your levels and get to an exercise that you can't do, just skip over it and come back later. I guarantee that in time everything will come together. Pilates makes sense for everybody — remember that it's magic!

If you have a neck or spinal injury, especially if the injury involves a vertebral disc problem, I recommend seeing an experienced Pilates practitioner trained in rehabilitation before trying Pilates at home. People who have suffered certain kinds of spinal injuries should not do many of the Pilates mat exercises. The mat series is designed for the healthy body, and exercises must be modified by a rehabilitation professional if a spinal injury is present.

Learning the Pilates Alphabet

Here's a list of the letters in the Pilates alphabet:

- Neutral Spine
- Abdominal Scoop
- Bridge
- C Curve: Lumbar, Thoracic, and Cervical
- Hip-Up
- Levitation
- Balance Point
- Stacking the Spine
- Pilates Abdominal Position
- Pilates First Position

The Pilates method has over 200 exercises, many of which are quite complicated and difficult to remember. The vast array of exercises can seem a little overwhelming at first. But almost every exercise contains basic movements that repeat over and over in the repertoire. When I started training teachers in the Pilates method, I realized that there must be a simple way to break down the exercises and make it easier for people to remember the repertoire. I thought long and hard and came up with what I now call the Pilates alphabet.

The Pilates alphabet is meant to facilitate the learning process and demystify even the most complex Pilates exercises by breaking them down into discrete and definable parts. Just as the English alphabet contains letters that together make up words, the Pilates alphabet contains basic movements and body concepts that constitute Pilates exercises. You find these Pilates alphabet "letters" in all Pilates exercises.

So, the Pilates alphabet is not a universal concept, but a personal, Ellie Herman-esque concept. Only I, my teachers, and now you know this alphabet, so don't expect all Pilates trainers to use this lingo. You're now privy to what only the highly privileged knew before. Whatever! The important thing is that if you walk into a Pilates studio, you need to know that the trainers there won't be using the alphabet that I use throughout this book — although they probably will have some other way of talking about basic movements.

Because the elements of the Pilates alphabet are so important, I'm asking you to pull out your mat (or just clear some space on your rug) and introduce yourself to them.

Neutral Spine

Neutral Spine is one of the most subtle yet powerful principles in the Pilates alphabet. It belongs to the less-is-more approach to movement, like most of the fundamental concepts underlying the Pilates method.

Here's how you can feel Neutral Spine: Lie on your back with your knees bent and your feet flat on the floor. Your spine should have two areas that do not touch the mat underneath you: your neck and your lower back (the cervical spine and lumbar spine, respectively). These natural curves in your back function to absorb shock when you're standing, running, jumping, or simply walking around town. When you sit, it's important to maintain the natural curves in your spine to prevent lower back and neck strain. Neutral Spine is basically universal proper posture.

More about Neutral Spine

When lying on your back with Neutral Spine, you should be able to balance a teacup on your lower belly. If you tilt your pelvis forward too much (by arching your back off the mat), your teacup will spill forward. This is called anterior pelvic tilt. If you tilt your pelvis backward (by flattening your back on the floor), you'll spill your teacup backward. This is called posterior pelvic tilt. Neutral Spine (also sometimes called neutral pelvis) is when the teacup doesn't spill!

To get technical: *Neutral pelvis* is actually defined as the pubic bone and the hip bones being on the same plane. You can feel these bony landmarks with your fingers if you're lying down, and this triangle of bones, when neutral, should create a flat table for your teacup. When standing up, you want to translate this idea of neutral pelvis to the upright position. When you're standing, the plane (or tabletop) created by the neutral pelvis should be perpendicular to the floor; you don't want your pubic bone pointing forward or back, but dropping straight down to the ground. Many people have the tendency to tilt their pelvis in one direction or the other, and either of these postural habits can cause strain to the body over time. Neutral Spine and neutral pelvis are just simply good posture, and when you have good posture, your muscles don't have to work so hard to keep you upright and moving.

You often work in Neutral Spine when performing stability exercises in Pilates in order to maintain and reinforce these natural curves in the spine. Many people are taught to flatten the curve of their lower back when doing exercises or when standing. This method is no longer thought to be posturally correct; instead, the natural curve is indicated. Figures 3-1a and 3-1b show the back with too much curve and not enough curve, respectively. Figure 3-1c shows true Neutral Spine. Note that Neutral Spine can be called for even when you're not on your back — some of the exercises in Chapter 10 call for Neutral Spine when you're on all fours, for example.

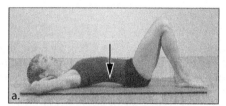 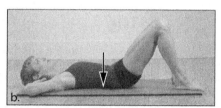

Too much curve (anterior pelvic tilt)...   not enough curve (posterior pelvic tilt)...

Figure 3-1:
Finding
Neutral
Spine.

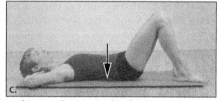

and just right (neutral pelvis).

Abdominal Scoop

You can do the Abdominal Scoop in any position, anywhere, anytime. It is easy and fun to do in your spare time, and it hides your spare tire! Basically, it's the act of pulling your navel in toward your spine. Imagining that you're zipping up a tight pair of pants or sucking in your gut will do the job.

What you're doing, anatomically, is engaging your deepest abdominal muscle (called your *tranversus abdominis*), which functions to hold your viscera in and, when contracted, decreases the diameter of the abdominal wall. When pulled taut, it works a lot like a drawstring around a pair of sweat pants. The reason you scoop in Pilates is that your deep abdominals help to stabilize your back and tend to be weak in most people. The superficial abdominal muscle *(rectus abdominis),* on the other hand, tends to be a workaholic and takes over the work of the deeper layers if you're not careful. So keep reminding your belly to pull in! Figure 3-2 shows the Abdominal Scoop in action.

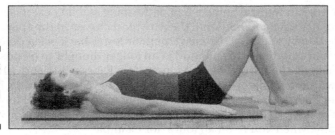

Figure 3-2:
The
Abdominal
Scoop.

Bridge

The Bridge is both a position and an exercise. (See Chapter 5 for the exercise.) Lie on your back with your knees bent and your feet flat on the floor. Push your hips up and hold them there. Take a deep breath in, and as you exhale, squeeze the butt, drop the rib cage, and pull your navel in toward your spine to make your torso as flat as possible. Your body should make a flat plane, with no bowing of the body up or down. You can maintain this tabletop torso by continuing to squeeze your butt and knitting your rib cage down into your belly. You'll feel a good burn in the back of your legs *(hamstrings)* and in your butt *(gluteus)*. Figure 3-3 shows the position.

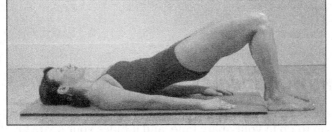

Figure 3-3:
The Bridge
position.

C Curve

The modern dance maven Martha Graham revolutionized dance by developing the concept of rounding the back (the Graham contraction). Before her, ballet dancers kept the spine always erect, ethereal, and lifted up off of this gravity-laden planet called Earth. Joe Pilates trained Ms. Graham at his New York Studio, and they must have shared some champagne (champagne is a Pilates tradition in the New York old school) and contractions in some of their sessions because the C Curve is a basic shape in the Pilates repertoire. The C Curve is a movement of the spine that strengthens the deep abdominals while stretching the muscles of the back.

The classic C Curve is always initiated by the abdominals. Try a C Curve by sitting up tall with your legs slightly bent in front of you. Imagine someone punching you in the lower stomach, and allow your spine to round by scooping in your deep abdominals. Your upper back, neck, and head may naturally follow this motion and round forward. So you initiate the C Curve with the lower back *(lumbar spine),* then you add the upper back *(thoracic spine),* and finally you add the head and neck *(cervical spine).* Now your whole spine is making a capital C. This movement should feel like a big stretch for your whole spine and all the muscles that surround it.

Here's a little more specific information about the three natural curves of the spine and how they participate in the C Curve movement.

Lumbar C Curve

The Lumbar C Curve movement is always initiated by your lower abdominals. This is the most difficult spinal movement to initiate because the lumbar spine has thick vertebrae that are meant to stabilize and hold the weight of the body. When you're standing or lying, the natural curve of your lumbar spine is in slight extension (like Neutral Spine), so when performing a Lumbar C Curve, you must pay much attention to pulling in your abdominals from the lowest part of your abdomen and attempting to reverse the natural curve of your low spine. You can accomplish this only by deep and strong low abdominal engagement. Figure 3-4 shows the Lumbar C Curve.

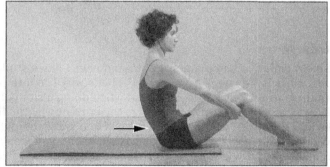

Figure 3-4:
The Lumbar
C Curve.

Thoracic C Curve

The upper back (thoracic region) naturally curves forward in a C shape (at least with most people — longtime dancers and gymnasts can develop a flattened or reverse thoracic curve from years of sticking out their chest). When performing a Thoracic C Curve, think of pulling your ribs in and allowing your shoulders to round forward, as in Figure 3-5. Doing so creates a nice stretch in the upper back.

The Thoracic C Curve naturally follows the Lumbar C Curve, but it is easy to do the Thoracic C Curve without actually starting from the lower back. In other words, it's easy for people to round their upper back because the back naturally rounds in that direction. Initiating the rounding from the lower back is more difficult and takes low abdominal work. The idea in Pilates is generally to try to do more work from the belly and to move the spine starting from the lower back and then adding in the upper back afterward. Be aware that you may have a tendency to just hunch forward like Quasimodo when doing a C Curve and round only from your upper back without actually using your low belly!

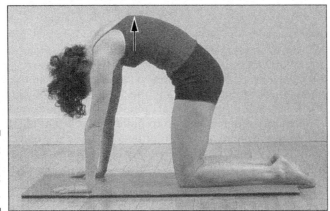

Figure 3-5:
The
Thoracic C
Curve.

Cervical C Curve

One of the most common complaints I get from novice Pilates students after their first mat class is "My neck bothers me!" That's why I go into painstaking detail about the correct way to lift your head when doing a sit-up. I use the Cervical C Curve mostly as a way to visualize the correct way to lift your head off the mat during an abdominal exercise. If you know the right way to lift your head up and understand proper neck alignment, you won't over-strain your neck when doing the abdominal-related exercises in Pilates.

Lie on your back with your hands interlaced behind your head to support the neck. Lift your head off the mat by lengthening the back of the neck and by imagining that you're squeezing a tangerine under your chin to bring the head up (kind of like nodding your head yes as you lift it off the mat). Don't lead up with your chin. Once your head is off the mat, you have created your Cervical C Curve; the C shape begins at the top of your head and ends at the base of your sternum (or rib cage). You must lift your head high enough to form the shape of the C. Think of your abdominal muscles lifting up the weight of the head, not the neck muscles. If you're very tight in your neck or very weak in your tummy, you may not be able to make a complete C shape. But if you keep doing the work, you will! Figure 3-6 shows a Cervical C Curve.

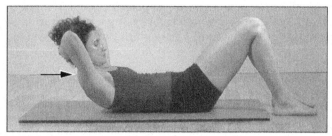

Figure 3-6:
The Cervical
C Curve.

Hip-Up

The Hip-Up is both part of the Pilates alphabet and a fundamental exercise. The name says it all. Lie on your back with your legs up, your knees bent and your feet crossed, and your arms down by your sides. Rock back and lift your hips up by using your low Abdominal Scoop. The Hip-Up can be very challenging for those with a weak tummy, a tight back, or a large lower body! For more details about how to do the Hip-Up, see Chapter 4. Figure 3-7 shows a Hip-Up.

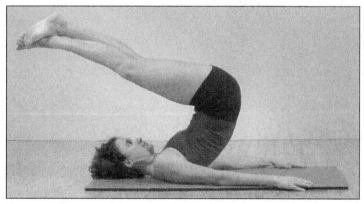

Figure 3-7:
Hip-Up.

Levitation

When you combine a Hip-Up with a little low butt squeeze, you get Levitation. If you lie on your back and lift up your hips with your Abdominal Scoop, and then at the top of the Hip-Up you squeeze your butt, you'll feel your hips levitate, rising perceptively higher as if the hand of a goddess came down and lifted you from the heavens. Levitation is a key concept in Pilates, but don't feel intimidated by Figure 3-8, which is an example of Levitation — you won't have to do anything like that until you get into the more advanced exercises.

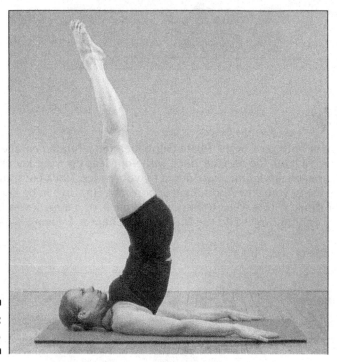

Figure 3-8:
Levitation.

Balance Point

Balance Point is both a position and a fundamental exercise. You can practice Balance Point by sitting up with your knees bent and holding onto the backs of your thighs. Then roll back slightly behind your tailbone, pull your belly in (your Abdominal Scoop, from earlier in this chapter), and lift your feet off the mat. In order to maintain your balance and stop yourself from rolling backward, you must engage and pull in your deep abdominal muscles. This position pulls you into your Lumbar C Curve (another letter of the Pilates alphabet!) and teaches you that to balance with ease, you must engage your deep center. Chapter 4 has detailed instructions for performing the Balance Point exercise, and Figure 3-9 gives you an idea of what Balance Point looks like.

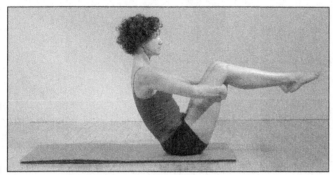

Figure 3-9:
Balance
Point.

Stacking the Spine

Stacking the Spine is a finish to several exercises in the Pilates method. It teaches *articulation* of the spine (full movement throughout all the vertebrae) as well as how to sit up vertically. It's a fluid way to sit up or stand erect from a hunched-over position. Also, Stacking the Spine is a wonderful stretch for your back. Figure 3-10 shows Stacking the Spine in action.

To practice Stacking the Spine, start by sitting with your knees bent and your feet on the floor. If this is a difficult position for you because you're tight in your hips or low back, then sit on a pillow. Allow your whole spine to round forward, letting your head hang heavy. Then begin to Stack the Spine by pulling your navel in toward your spine. Start at the lowest vertebra possible, moving up one vertebra at a time and allowing your head to hang heavy until the end. Finally, you're sitting up tall. You have just Stacked your Spine! You can try again, but this time try reversing the stacking to get to the starting point. In other words, allow your head to initiate the roll down and then move one vertebra at a time until you're rounded forward (in a C Curve) and are ready to stack up again. If you're having trouble feeling where your vertical is, try Stacking the Spine with your back against the wall.

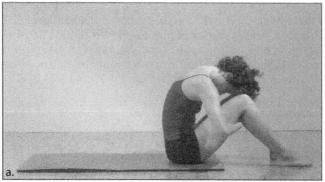

Move your back one vertebra at a time.

Figure 3-10:
Stacking the
Spine.

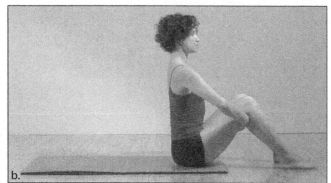

Pilates Abdominal Position

Pilates Abdominal Position is a name I came up with to describe the place-ment of the upper body when performing the lion's share of Pilates abdomi-nal exercises. Using the Cervical C Curve described earlier in this chapter, lie on your back and lift your head off the mat just high enough that your shoul-der blades are just off the mat; you can imagine that the base of your sternum is anchored down to the floor and the back of your neck is lengthening. Figure 3-11 shows the Pilates Abdominal Position.

Maintaining this position is essential when performing abdominal exercises. If you allow the head to drop back, you'll begin to feel fatigue in the neck, and you won't be using your abdominals as much. The upper abdominals should be working to maintain this position (and that's where you should feel the burn). Again, if you're very tight in your neck or upper back, holding the Pilates abdominal position will be very difficult. Don't give up! Many people have a hard time with this, so just do the best you can, and eventually you'll loosen up. You still get the benefits of the exercise even if you're not able to come all the way up to the classic Pilates Abdominal Position.

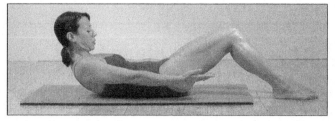

Figure 3-11:
Pilates
Abdominal
Position.

Pilates First Position

A ballet dancer standing in first position has her legs together and turned out from the hip, her knees facing away from each other, and her feet making a V shape. In Pilates, First Position is very much the same: You turn out your hips and make a small V shape, with your heels squeezing together (see Figure 3-12). You never want to force the turn-out. Simply get in a comfortable position, with your knees facing away from each other and your inner thighs squeezing together. You use this Pilates First Position in many exercises instead of keeping your legs parallel. Turning out from the hips engages the inner thigh muscles and the low butt, which we like to use as much as possible in Pilates. Pilates First Position refers just to what the legs are doing in relation to each other. You can be in the position when you're standing, lying down, and so on.

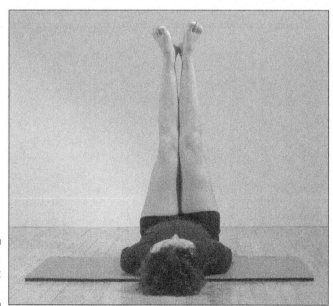

Figure 3-12:
Pilates First
Position.

Turn your legs out from the hips.

Don't believe everything I say!

Here's a good place to make a large disclaimer. But first, an anecdote. During a trip to Oregon, I met up with an old friend who also happens to be a master Pilates teacher. We spent time doing what all Pilates instructors love to do when they get together: talking about the intricacies of the body and how to better teach the method. My friend admits, like all good teachers do, that not one position, or one rule, works for everybody. The more experience you have teaching different bodies, the more you realize that there is no such thing as one right position or one right cue that is universal.

In the case of the Pilates Abdominal Position, for instance, ideally you want to be able to roll up off the mat with your upper body to the point where the bottom edge of your shoulder blades are just off the mat. But some people have huge shoulder blades, and others have tiny ones. Some people have extremely tight upper backs or flattened curves in their upper backs, making it impossible to roll up to this point. So this rule works only for the average Jane who has average-size shoulder blades and a flexible upper back. Please take this disclaimer into account with all the rules and "letters" of the alphabet. If your body doesn't do a certain thing I describe, make a mental note of it. I describe ideals to strive toward, but not necessarily achieve. I try to mention what types of issues limit your ability to reach the ideal. Some of these limitations are things you can't change (such as limitations resulting from your bone structure), while other limitations will definitely fade away with practice and conditioning. You need to know what the ideal is for the average person, but each person needs to develop her own definition of "ideal" to fit her own body. One of the most important aspects of Pilates is learning about your body and what makes it different from the norm, and striving for your own individual ideal.

Part II
Mat Exercises

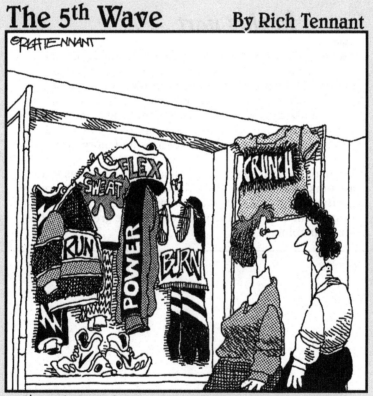

The 5th Wave   By Rich Tennant

"I'm not sure I can live up to my workout clothes."

In this part . . .

The exercises in the mat series are the heart of Pilates. In this part, I take you through four different series: pre-Pilates, beginning, intermediate, and advanced. If you're a Pilates novice, start with the pre-Pilates series so that your body can get used to the challenging movements that make up Pilates. As you move up to the advanced series, you do more difficult exercises and more of them.

In Chapters 8 through 10, I present some exercises that are outside the series. Read these chapters if you're ready for the really hard stuff, want some extra exercises that target your butt and thighs, or want some great stretches for your spine.

Chapter 4

Pre-Pilates: The Fundamentals

In This Chapter

▶ Getting your body ready for real Pilates moves

▶ Understanding the fundamental movements and exercises

*T*he exercises in this chapter are sometimes called pre-Pilates because they are preparations to get your body ready to do the harder stuff. These are definitely what you should do when you're first introducing yourself to Pilates, and then you can do them in the future as a warm-up for the more advanced exercises. And you can always come back to these basics, no matter how advanced you get, to refresh your form.

Practice this fundamental series until you understand these basic concepts in both your body and your mind, and then move on to the beginning series.

I include some of these fundamental exercises in the beginning and intermediate series. I think that the Upper Abdominal Curls and Coccyx Curls are two exercises that are always great to start your workout. Why? Well, Coccyx Curls warm up your lower back and get you connected to your deep abdominals, while the Upper Abdominal Curls warm up your neck and upper back and get you feeling that Pilates Abdominal Position.

When doing this series of exercises, be aware of the sensations in your body. If you really get the concept that the exercise is trying to teach, then you may not need to repeat it the next time you work out. Ultimately, the goal is to incorporate these concepts in the more advanced series and be able to build more complex movement phrases.

In this book, I try to give you as much help as possible by giving you a set of exercises that match whatever level you're at. The fundamentals are in this chapter, Chapter 5 has beginning exercises, and so on. Do the exercises in the order that they're presented in each series, because this order makes sense for your body. And don't feel bad about progressing slowly! Start here, stick with the program, and eventually you'll be doing the Boomerang with the best of 'em.

One other thing: The models in this book are all experienced Pilates instructors. Don't feel like you need to look like them, exactly, as you perform the exercise. Their form is something to strive for, but don't expect yourself to match it perfectly.

A Word of Caution

Before you get started doing Pilates, I want to take a second to remind you to please be careful. If you injure yourself while exercising, you're hurting your health, not improving it!

Here are some signs that an exercise isn't right for you:

- You feel a sharp, shooting, or tingling pain while exercising.
- You feel a muscle pulling while doing an exercise, and the pain doesn't subside in a few minutes.
- Your neck hurts while doing an exercise.
- One or more of your joints hurt while doing an exercise.

Your lower back may feel sensations when doing Pilates, but that may not be a bad thing. Bad back pain is the kind that doesn't go away after a few minutes but lasts for days afterward. If you feel your back hurting when doing an abdominal exercise, you must modify it until you don't feel your back anymore. Usually you just need to pull your navel in a lot more! As your abdominal muscles get stronger, your back will stop bothering you.

The Series in This Chapter

Here's a preview of the series in this chapter:

- Breathing in Neutral Spine
- Shoulder Shrugs
- Shoulder Slaps
- Arm Reaches/Arm Circles
- Coccyx Curls
- Tiny Steps
- Upper Abdominal Curls

✔ Hip-Up

✔ C Curve Roll Down Prep

✔ Balance Point/Teaser Prep

✔ Rolling Like a Ball, Modified

Breathing in Neutral Spine

Most people don't breathe into the lower portions of their lungs, but only breathe superficially. This exercise focuses on increasing lung capacity and especially on bringing air into the deeper parts of the lung.

Breathing is something we all do automatically, and yet some people tend to hold their breath when exercising. Holding your breath tenses your muscles and makes your body more rigid. Even though the following exercise may seem unbearably easy, it's actually the fundamental essence that underlies all future Pilates exercises.

Getting set

Lie down on your back with your knees bent and your feet flat on the floor about hip distance apart. Relax your back into Neutral Spine (see Chapter 3). Place your hands on either side of your lower rib cage just above your waist, putting your thumbs toward your back and your other fingers toward your breastbone.

The exercise

Inhale: Breathe deeply into your lungs, allowing your ribs to expand laterally in your hands. Think of breathing into your kidney area (your lower back) and filling up your lungs to their fullest capacity. Try not to arch your back off the mat at all.

Exhale: Allow all the air to come out of your lungs, as you pull your navel in toward your spine.

You are playing an accordion. As you inhale, the squeeze box expands open; as you exhale, it comes back together.

Do's and don'ts

✔ Don't arch your back when you inhale. Keep your upper back in contact with the mat.

✔ Do continue this exercise until you feel relaxed and grounded and ready to proceed with the next exercise.

Shoulder Shrugs

Feeling uptight? Tension is a physical as well as an emotional reality. Most people unknowingly hold tension in their neck and shoulders, especially if they work at a computer or have a desk job. Not overusing your *upper trapezius muscles* (the muscles at the back of your neck and at the top of your shoulders) is almost impossible if you hold your arms in front of you hour after hour. But once you become aware of this holding pattern you can correct it through this simple exercise.

Getting set

To begin, lie down on your back with your knees bent, your feet flat on the floor about hip distance apart, and your arms straight down by your sides. Relax your back into Neutral Spine.

The exercise

Inhale: Bring your shoulders up by your ears, contracting your upper trapezius muscles (Figure 4-1).

Exhale: Relax and release your shoulders, letting them drop down quickly away from the ears.

Complete 4 repetitions. On the final repetition, slow down and, on the exhale, let your shoulder blades melt slowly down your back. Try to feel the muscles in your back that keep the shoulder blades down and away from your ears.

Do's and don'ts

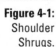

- ✔ Do follow the breathing cues in this exercise. Exhaling always helps relax your muscles.

- ✔ Don't hold your breath.

Figure 4-1:
Shoulder
Shrugs.

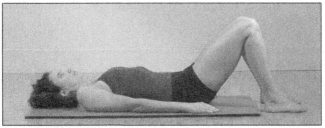

Shrug, then release, your shoulders.

Shoulder Slaps

Shoulder Slaps are another safe and simple way to discover how to relax and release your shoulder muscles as well as a way to discover how to engage the stabilizing muscles of your shoulder.

Getting set

Lying on your back with your knees bent and your feet flat on the floor, bring your arms up so that your fingers point toward the ceiling.

The exercise

Inhale: Reach your arms up to the sky, allowing your shoulder blades *(scapulae)* to come off the mat (Figure 4-2).

Exhale: Keep your arms straight and reach up as you relax and release your shoulder muscles, letting your scapulae slap back to the mat.

Complete 4 repetitions.

On the final repetition, allow your shoulder blades to return slowly, imagining your shoulder blades melting back into the mat. Keep pushing your scapulae back into the mat, and feel the muscles that are working — these are your *latissimus dorsi muscles.* It is important to know where the latissimus dorsi muscles are because you use them all the time in Pilates to pull your shoulders down away from your ears, helping to release shoulder tension.

Do's and don'ts

✔ Do really release on the exhale, allowing your shoulder blades and arms to truly drop with gravity.

✔ Don't bend your arms when you slap the shoulder blades down.

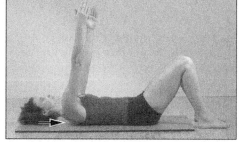

Figure 4-2:
Shoulder
Slaps.

Lift your shoulders off the mat.

Arm Reaches/Arm Circles

This exercise has the dual function of stretching out the chest and back muscles while teaching upper torso stability.

If you are tight and need to stretch, focus on opening your chest when performing this exercise. If you are a noodle and have lots of flexibility in your body, then focus on stabilizing your torso. (Don't let your upper back arch off the mat!)

Getting set

Lie on your back with your knees bent and your feet flat on the floor, approximately hip distance apart, and your back in Neutral Spine, arms down by your sides.

The exercise

Inhale: Reach your arms up to the ceiling at a 90-degree angle to the floor, keeping your arms shoulder distance apart (Figure 4-3a).

Exhale: Drop your rib cage and think of knitting your ribs into your belly, and reach your arms back toward your ears (Figure 4-3b). Use your upper abdominals to keep your upper back from arching off the mat. Figure 4-4 shows incorrect posture, with the back arched off the mat.

Inhale: Circle the arms open to a T shape (keeping the arms on the floor, as in Figure 4-3c), then down by your sides and then back to the starting position, reaching up to the sky.

Complete 3 repetitions and reverse directions.

Do's and don'ts

- ✔ Do maintain absolute stability in your torso by keeping your ribs down.

- ✔ Do keep your shoulders down away from your ears as you initiate the exercise.

- ✔ Don't let your upper back arch off the mat (Figure 4-4). As you raise your arms, your upper back naturally wants to go with them — the whole point of this exercise is to keep your back on the mat.

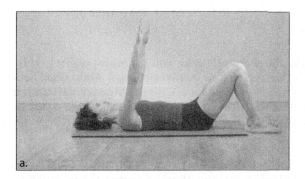

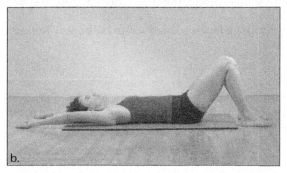

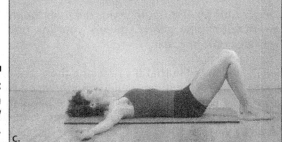

Figure 4-3:
Arm
Reaches/
Arm Circles.

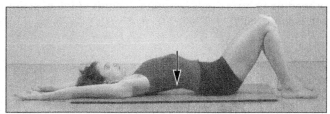

Figure 4-4:
What not to
do when
performing
Arm
Reaches/
Arm Circles.

Don't allow your back to arch off the mat.

Coccyx Curls

Now that your shoulders are released, you can move down to the center of it all. This is your first exercise that involves the low Abdominal Scoop that is so prevalent in Pilates exercises. Please don't allow your shoulders to rise and hold tension now that you've got some release there — just because you're not focusing on the shoulders doesn't mean that you get to go back to bad habits!

In this exercise, you learn through movement the three most basic parts of the Pilates alphabet: Neutral Spine, the Abdominal Scoop, and Bridge.

Coccyx, by the way, is just a fancy name for the tailbone. "Tailbone Curl" just doesn't sound as good.

Getting set

Lie on your back with your knees bent and your feet flat on the floor, approximately hip distance apart, and your back in Neutral Spine, arms down by your sides (Figure 4-5a).

The exercise

Inhale: Breathe in deeply.

Exhale: Begin the Coccyx Curl by first finding your deep Abdominal Scoop: Pull your navel in toward your spine, gently squeeze your low butt muscles, and flatten your lower back onto the mat.

Imagine that your belly is so pulled in that it's pressing the vertebrae of the lower back onto the mat. This is sometimes called *imprinting* because you're picturing yourself imprinting your vertebrae onto the mat beneath you with your Abdominal Scoop. If you were lying on a beach and pressing your low back onto the sand with your Abdominal Scoop, you would see an imprint of the vertebrae on the sand afterward. If the imprinting image doesn't work for you, imagine that you have to zip up a very tight pair of pants.

If the two preceding images don't get you to scoop, think of scooping out a melon, which is your belly!

Inhale: Release and go back to a comfortable Neutral Spine.

Exhale: Find your Abdominal Scoop again by pulling your navel in toward your spine and gently squeezing your low butt muscles. Flatten your lower back onto the mat and then keep rolling your tailbone slowly up off the mat to the count of 5. Roll up to the Bridge position (Figure 4-5b). Your body should make a straight line from your shoulders to your knees. Don't press your hips up so high that you can't see your knees.

Inhale: Hold the Bridge position.

Exhale: Roll down one vertebra at a time, again by pulling in your belly. Return to Neutral Spine at the end.

Complete 3 repetitions, each time making the movement smaller and smaller until on the last one you're not even moving out of Neutral Spine, but are pulling your abdominals in as if you were going to initiate a Coccyx Curl but don't. This is called engaged Neutral Spine. See the sidebar "Why engaged Neutral Spine is so important" for more info.

Do's and don'ts

✔ Do focus on initiating this movement with the Abdominal Scoop.

✔ Don't tense your upper body when doing this exercise. Keep your neck long and your shoulders relaxed.

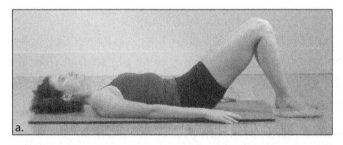

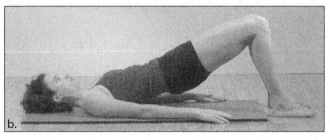

Figure 4-5:
Coccyx
Curls.

Why engaged Neutral Spine is so important

If you carry over engaged Neutral Spine to standing up, you will have the beginnings of very good posture. It allows you to keep the natural curves of the spine while still having deep abdominal engagement to support your back. Engaged Neutral Spine on the mat simply means your belly is pulled in but you have not changed the position of your pelvis on the mat. To make sure you are in Neutral Spine, keep your tailbone in contact with the mat.

Tiny Steps

Tiny Steps is a stability exercise that tests the strength and stability of your lower abdominals. You want to keep Neutral Spine throughout Tiny Steps but at the same time really use your Abdominal Scoop. The point of this exercise is to not move your hips or your lower back while moving your legs up and down. It looks simple, but it actually takes quite a bit of inner strength (of the muscle variety). You're going for absolute stability here!

Getting set

Lie down on your back with your knees bent and your feet flat on the floor about hip distance apart. Relax your back into Neutral Spine. Put your hands on your hip bones so that you can feel whether you're moving or rocking from side to side (Figure 4-6a).

The exercise

Exhale: Pull your navel in toward your spine and lift your right knee up to your chest (Figure 4-6b).

Inhale: Hold the position.

Exhale: Pull your navel in toward your spine, and bring your right leg back down to the mat, controlling the movement from the center and returning to the starting position.

Alternate legs, and complete 8 repetitions.

Do's and don'ts

 ✔ Don't let your lower back arch or your hips rock side to side.

 ✔ Don't tense your upper body when doing this exercise. Keep your neck long and your shoulders relaxed.

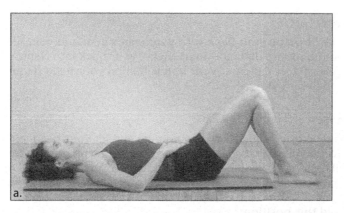

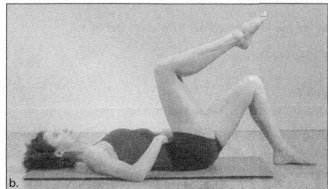

Figure 4-6:
Tiny Steps.

Upper Abdominal Curls

This exercise may be hard for you for two reasons:

- ✔ If you have weak upper abdominal muscles, you'll shake when attempting to roll up. Don't worry too much if you can't come up in this curl; you'd be surprised how many people have a hard time with this exercise at first.

- ✔ If you have a very tight upper back and neck, you may not be able to get into the position. If this is the case, then it will be virtually impossible for you to come up, and you may or may not feel any work in your abdominal muscles. You will, however feel a stretch in the back of your neck and upper back.

In either case, keep trying. If you get frustrated, just move on to the next exercise and revisit this one after a few weeks of other Pilates exercises. You'll slowly transform, and you may find this one easier at a future date.

Getting set

To begin, lie down on your back with your knees bent and your feet flat on the floor about hip distance apart. Relax your back into Neutral Spine. Interlace your fingers and put your hands behind your head (Figure 4-7a). Take a deep breath in.

The exercise

Exhale: Pull your navel in toward your spine and lift your head, pulling your chin in toward your chest as if you are squeezing a tangerine under your chin, as you roll up to your Pilates Abdominal Position. You should roll up just high enough that your shoulder blades are barely off the mat, as in Figure 4-7.

Inhale: Hold this position.

Exhale: Control the movement back down to the mat.

Complete 8 slow repetitions.

Do's and don'ts

- ✔ Do maintain Neutral Spine as you roll up.
- ✔ Don't let your lower back flatten; keep your tailbone anchored to the mat.
- ✔ Don't strain your neck. Allow your hands to hold the weight of your head and keep the space of a tangerine between your chin and your neck.

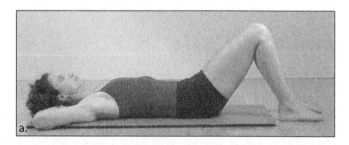

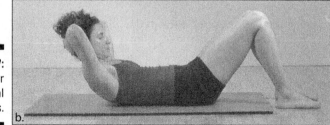

Figure 4-7:
Upper
Abdominal
Curls.

Hip-Up

The Hip-Up is a preliminary exercise and a part of the Pilates alphabet. By lifting your hips, you strengthen your lower abdominal muscles (and your butt muscles as well, if you squeeze your butt on the way up).

If you have a neck injury, proceed with caution. Skip this exercise if it causes any strain on your neck.

If you feel that your neck and shoulders are tensing too much, try putting your arms above your head. Doing so takes your upper body out of the movement and accentuates your abdominals. If you don't have sufficient abdominal strength, you will need to keep your arms down by your sides to assist you in lifting your hips.

Getting set

Lie on your back with your legs bent and up in the air and your feet crossed. Have your arms down by your sides with your palms facing down (Figure 4-8a).

The exercise

Inhale: Rock back and pull your navel in toward your spine as you lift your hips off the mat (Figure 4-8b). Press your palms and upper arms into the mat to help lift yourself up. Keep your shoulders and neck relaxed. Start very small. Use the momentum of your legs reaching back to help you create the rocking movement.

Exhale: Control the lowering of your hips by pulling in your belly, again using your arms as needed.

Complete 9 repetitions. You can try raising your hips a little higher each time. Make sure you never roll up so high that you roll onto your neck. On the last one, try rolling all the way back up to sitting so that you can easily transition to C Curve Roll Down Prep, the next exercise.

Do's and don'ts

- ✔ Do remember that this is a lower abdominal exercise, so use your arms to help you get your butt up, but only as much as you need to. Focus on doing most of the work with your belly.

- ✔ Do think of a creating a rocking motion that is smooth in both directions. Think of massaging your spine as you roll up and down.

- ✔ Don't lift your hips straight up to the sky, but think of aiming your hips over your head, creating a circular motion rather than an up-and-down motion.

✔ Don't roll back too far, or you'll roll onto your fragile cervical vertebrae (your neck!) and potentially cause neck problems. Think of keeping your neck long and relaxed.

Modification

As you get stronger, try making the exercise more challenging. Do 3 repetitions lifting up just your butt, 3 more going a little higher by lifting up to your middle back, and the last 3 rolling up to your upper back. On the last 3 highest ones, squeeze your butt at the top of the Hip-Up and feel the weight of your hips Levitate off the floor (Levitation is a letter of the Pilates alphabet, which I explain in Chapter 3).

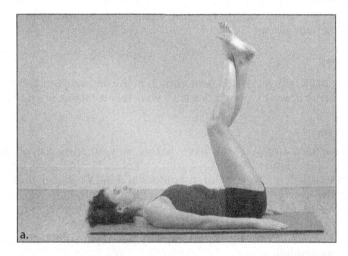

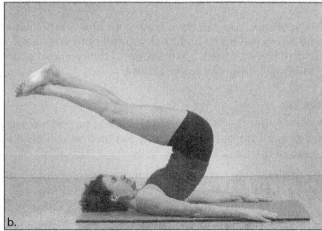

Figure 4-8: Hip-Up.

C Curve Roll Down Prep

Now you're getting into the fun stuff. This exercise is a preparation for Roll Down, which is a preparation for Roll Up! You may be strong enough already to do a full Roll Up. If so, you will progress quickly through this series and the next. But, if you have little awareness of your deep abdominals and little strength, plan on taking things slowly and know that you are in the majority.

Ultimately, one of the most satisfying things about Pilates is that it is challenging — take up the challenge, and you'll feel great as you slowly conquer more and more difficult exercises.

C Curve Roll Down Prep — the name is pretty self-explanatory. You guide yourself as you become aware of how to feel your C Curve in your lower back. You also get some practice with Stacking the Spine. (C Curve and Stacking the Spine are both letters of the Pilates alphabet. See Chapter 3 for more information.)

Getting set

Sitting up, bend your knees and put your feet flat on the floor. Hold the back of your thighs with your hands, wrapping them around the outside of your legs (Figure 4-9a). Sit up as tall as you can by imagining you have a golden string attached to the back of the top of your head that is pulling you up to the sky.

The exercise

Inhale: Breathe in deeply and continue to sit up as tall as you can.

Exhale: Pull your navel in toward your spine and hollow out your low belly, making a C Curve shape in your low back. Imagine that someone punched you in your low belly. Begin rolling backward down your spine, allowing your tailbone to roll underneath you. Allow your arms to walk slowly down your thighs as needed and use your arms to assist you in the roll down. Try to roll far enough down that you can feel the bones of your lower back pressing onto the mat. Your whole back, including your neck and your head, should look like a big C. Figures 4-9b and 4-9c show the model rolling down.

Inhale: Take in a breath at the bottom.

Exhale: Pull your navel in toward your spine and think of pressing your lower back into the mat with your abdominal muscles as you slowly roll back up. Again, use your arms to assist you and allow them to walk back up your thighs. Allow your whole back to stay round in a C Curve and your belly to stay hollow as you return to sitting on your tailbone. You should be making a C shape with your whole spine (Figure 4-9d).

Inhale: Stack up the Spine, starting from your lower back, then your upper back, and then your head and neck. Think of keeping your head hanging heavy until the very end.

Exhale: Keep sitting up tall and allow your shoulders to drop down away from your ears. Feel the upper back muscles engage as they keep the shoulders down in their proper place (Figure 4-9e).

Complete 6 repetitions.

Do's and don'ts

- ✔ Do focus on using your abdominals to perform the exercise.
- ✔ Do attempt to articulate through your spine on the way down and on the way up.
- ✔ Do minimize the tension in your upper body; keep your neck long and relaxed.
- ✔ Don't hold your breath. Use long, slow breathing to assist the movement.

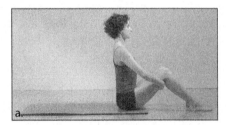 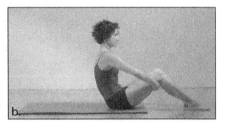

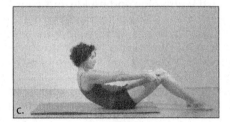 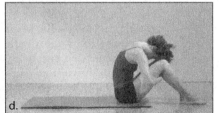

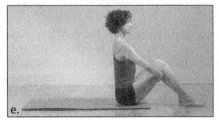

Figure 4-9:
C Curve Roll
Down Prep.

Balance Point/Teaser Prep

Balance Point is basically a C Curve Roll Down Prep with your feet off the floor. The fact that your feet are off the floor makes it much harder to keep your balance. If you find this exercise too daunting, simply practice the previous exercise until you're ready to progress.

Balance Point is both a fundamental exercise and a letter in the Pilates alphabet. Balance Point is one of the best exercises I know to find your deep abdominal muscles. You can't cheat and use other muscles to help out in this exercise; you are forced to use your deep abdominals because if you don't you'll fall out of position. This exercise really separates the women from the girls and the men from the boys.

In this exercise and in Pilates in general, articulating your spine is important. *Articulating* your spine means to move your spine one vertebra at a time, instead of moving the spine in chunks of four or five vertebrae. Articulating one vertebra at a time brings more flexibility to the spine and enables the abdominals to work more.

This exercise is also a good preparation for the more advanced exercise, the Teaser, which you encounter in Chapters 6 and 7.

Getting set

Sit up, bend your knees, and lift your feet off the floor, holding the back of your thighs with your hands (right hand wrapping around the outside of the right thigh and left hand around the outside of the left thigh). You should be balanced right behind your tailbone (coccyx), with your lower back rounded and your belly hollowed out (Figure 4-10a). This is the Balance Point position. Take a deep breath in.

The exercise

Exhale: Begin to roll down your spine, pushing your thighs away as a counterbalance. Pull your navel in and control the movement from the center. Only go back as far as you can control the movement (Figures 4-10b and 4-10c show the model rolling down).

Inhale: Maintain your position.

Exhale: Press your legs away and come back to the Balance Point position, using the hollow abdominal muscles to bring yourself back up.

Complete 6 repetitions. Attempt to increase the distance you go backward every time.

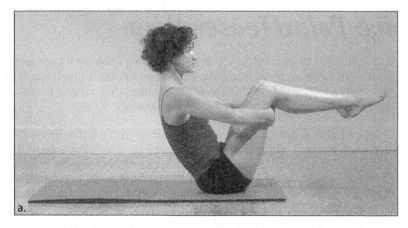

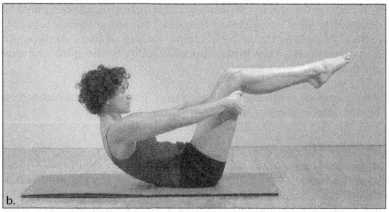

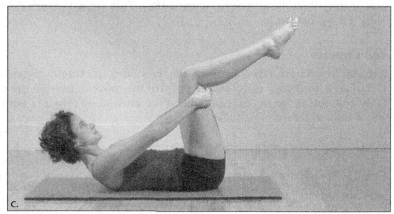

Figure 4-10:
Balance
Point/Teaser
Prep.

Do's and don'ts

✔ Do focus on using your abdominals to perform the exercise.

✔ Do attempt to articulate through your spine on the way down and on the way up.

✔ Do minimize the tension in your upper body; keep your neck long and relaxed.

✔ Don't overuse your arm muscles by heaving yourself up with your biceps.

Modifications

If this exercise is too hard for you to do and you keep falling backward, put your feet on the ground and proceed with the same instructions.

When you get the strength and control, you'll be able to go all the way to the floor and back up to the Balance Point. Once you've mastered that, try letting your arms free and allowing them to reach forward on the way down and on the way up. This is the beginning of the Teaser, versions of which are in Chapters 6 and 7.

Rolling Like a Ball, Modified

Rolling Like a Ball is a combination of Hip-Up and Balance Point. Combining both strength and control, this exercise is a fun way to massage your own back, find out how to articulate your spine, and find the abdominal control center.

This is the modified version because you are holding onto the thighs instead of onto the shins, as you do in the regular Rolling Like a Ball (Chapter 5). This modified handhold allows for more articulation and ease in the rolling movement because it allows more space between the thigh and the body.

If you have a neck injury, proceed with caution. Skip this exercise if it causes any strain in your neck.

Getting set

Start by sitting up in the same position as Balance Point (Figure 4-11a), with your legs bent and feet off the floor and your hands holding the back of your legs (right hand wrapping around the outside of the right thigh and left hand around the outside of the left thigh).

The exercise

Inhale: Roll back onto your upper back and do a Hip-Up, using your lower Abdominal Scoop to lift your hips, and squeeze your butt to get an extra lift (Figures 4-11b and 4-11c).

Exhale: Return to your Balance Point, using your Abdominal Scoop as the brake to the rolling (Figure 4-11d).

Do's and don'ts

- ✔ Do think of massaging your back by using your abdominals to help you articulate each vertebra.

- ✔ Do allow your momentum to help you roll backward, and control the movement with your abdominals at the top of the Hip-Up.

- ✔ Don't allow your back to make a thumping sound, especially on the way back up. Use your abdominals to pull into your lower back to make a smooth movement.

- ✔ Don't roll too far back onto your neck. If you don't have neck problems, you don't want to start having them now.

Modification

Rolling Like a Ball becomes more difficult the smaller the ball you make. If you hold your hands on the front of your knees, you tighten your ball, making this more of a control and abdominal exercise and less of a massage and articulation exercise.

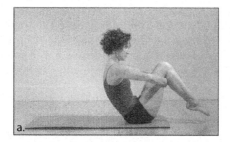
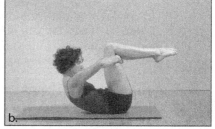

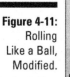

Figure 4-11:
Rolling
Like a Ball,
Modified.

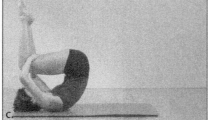
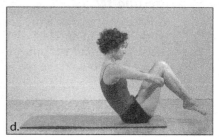

Return to the Balance Point.

Chapter 5

Now That You've Got the Basics Down: The Beginning Mat Series

In This Chapter

▶ Trying some actual Pilates exercises

▶ Beginning to feel the burn

*I*f you started your Pilates experience by doing the series in Chapter 4 (as I recommend), you've mastered what I call pre-Pilates exercises. You understand the fundamentals, both in your body and in your mind, so you're ready for a full-blown Pilates series.

Even the Hundred, which is the first new exercise in this series, requires a huge amount of upper abdominal strength and neck strength — so don't feel bad about having to take it slow and incorporating these exercises into your routine a little at a time. Before you move on to the next chapter, though, you should be able to move through this series fluidly and without much difficulty.

Just because you've mastered the pre-Pilates exercises doesn't mean that you should forget about them. In fact, I include a couple of the exercises from Chapter 4 (Coccyx Curls and Upper Abdominal Curls) as a warm-up for the series in this chapter so that your spine and your abdominals have a chance to get oiled up before launching into the Hundred. Then I include a couple additional exercises from Chapter 4, Balance Point and Hip-Up, because these movements are so important in Pilates.

The Series in This Chapter

Here are the exercises in the beginning series. Some of the exercises you've already done, assuming you've worked through the pre-Pilates exercises in Chapter 4. When this is the case, I include photos of the exercises in the text to remind you of the exercise, but I don't include a full description.

✔ Coccyx Curls (Chapter 4)

✔ Upper Abdominal Curls (Chapter 4)

✔ Hundred, Beginning Level

✔ Balance Point (Chapter 4)

✔ Hip-Up (Chapter 4)

✔ Rolling Like a Ball

✔ Single Leg Stretch

✔ Rising Swan

✔ Roll Down

✔ Bridge

✔ Spine Stretch Forward

✔ Side Kicks

Coccyx Curls

I like to start every workout with Coccyx Curls. They get your lower back warmed up and get you to feel your Abdominal Scoop. Coccyx Curls are shown in Figure 5-1 and are described in detail in Chapter 4. Complete 3 repetitions.

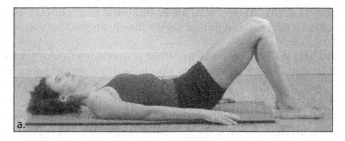

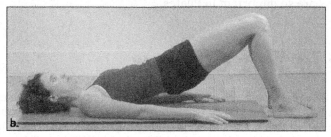

Figure 5-1:
Coccyx
Curls.

Upper Abdominal Curls

After doing Coccyx Curls, do Upper Abdominal Curls. I include this fundamental exercise as a warm-up for your upper back and neck and to get you to feel your Pilates Abdominal Position (when your shoulders are just off the mat). Upper Abdominal Curls are shown in Figure 5-2 and are described in detail in Chapter 4. Complete 8 slow repetitions.

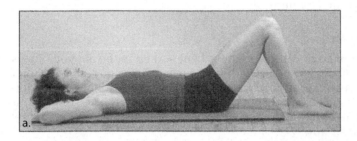

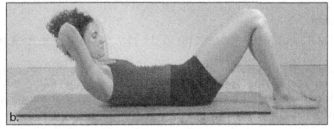

Figure 5-2:
Upper
Abdominal
Curls.

Hundred, Beginning Level

The Hundred got its name because you hold the exercise for 100 beats. It is a great exercise to come early in a series because it gets your whole body warm, possibly even breaking a sweat. It gets your breath going strong and your blood moving. In addition, the Hundred is an excellent exercise for increasing torso stability and abdominal strength. You may have some difficulty keeping your head up for so long. See the "Do's and don'ts" section for ways to protect your neck.

Getting set

Lie on your back with your knees bent and up in the air, your knees and hips forming 90-degree angles with your inner thighs squeezing together, in the tabletop position. Your back should be in Neutral Spine (see Chapter 3 for an explanation of Neutral Spine). Figure 5-3a shows the starting position. If this position feels like a strain on your lower back, try keeping your feet down on the floor for now.

The exercise

Inhale: Reach your arms straight up to the sky, palms facing forward.

Exhale: As you reach your arms back down to the floor, lift your head (think of squeezing a tangerine under your chin on the way up) and roll up to the Pilates Abdominal Position with your shoulder blades just off the mat. Your palms gently slap the floor in a percussive rhythm (Figure 5-3b).

Inhale: Inhale deeply for 5 beats (keep the rhythm with your arms), using accordion breathing.

Accordion breathing is *lateral chest breathing.* Imagine that your rib cage is an accordion. On the inhale, the accordion expands laterally, and on the exhale, the accordion squeezes back together.

Exhale: Using percussive breathing, exhale for 5 beats (saying shh, shh, shh, shh, shh).

Percussive breathing is forced exhalation using the abdominal muscles; think of forcing the air out in short percussive blows.

Hold the position and pulse your arms for 10 breaths (10 inhales and 10 exhales), so that they make 100 total beats.

Do's and don'ts

✔ Do remember that this is an abdominal exercise, not a neck exercise. You must be rolled up off the mat high enough to maximize the abdominal workout and minimize neck strain.

✔ Do press your lower back into your mat by using your Abdominal Scoop, especially on the exhale, maintaining your pelvis in its neutral position by keeping your tailbone grounded to the mat.

✔ Do think of reaching long away from yourself with your fingers and try to think of pulsing your arms from your back muscles, keeping your shoulder blades pulling down your back.

✔ Don't continue if your neck strains. Instead, put one hand behind the head to support the neck, and switch hands at 50 beats.

✔ Don't let yourself lose the Pilates Abdominal Position by sinking downward; accentuate the upper abdominal curl up on every exhale.

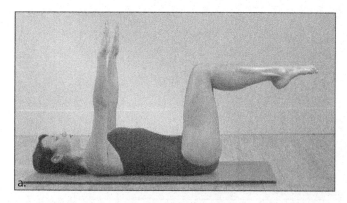

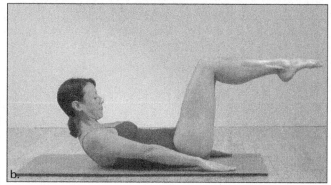

Figure 5-3:
Hundred, Beginning Level.

Balance Point/Teaser Prep

After doing the Hundred, do the Balance Point exercise from Chapter 4. See Figure 5-4 to refresh your memory. Complete 6 repetitions.

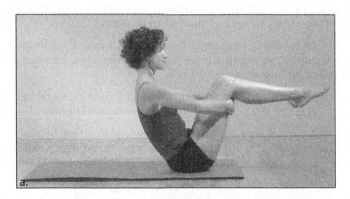

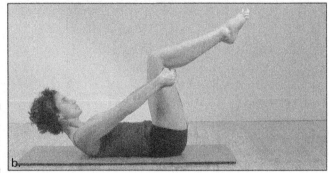

Figure 5-4:
Balance
Point.

Hip-Up

Hip-Up is the next exercise in the series. I describe it in detail in Chapter 4. Figure 5-5 shows you how it's done. Complete 9 repetitions.

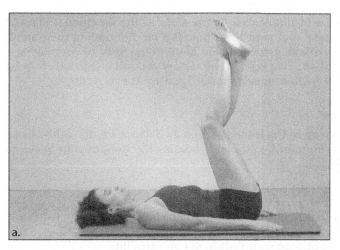

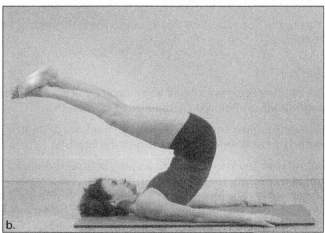

Figure 5-5:
Hip-Up.

Rolling Like a Ball

Rolling Like a Ball is a combination of Hip-Up and Balance Point. Requiring both strength and control, this exercise is a fun way to massage your own back, find out how to articulate your spine, and find abdominal control.

This exercise is almost exactly the same as the modified Rolling Like a Ball from Chapter 4, but your hand hold is a bit different. In this slightly more advanced version, your hands hold on to the front of your knees, keeping you in a tighter ball. This tighter ball makes you roll faster, which forces you to use your deep abdominals more to control the movement.

Getting set

Start sitting up in the same position as Balance Point, with your legs bent and off the floor and your hands holding the front of your knees (one hand on each knee).

The exercise

Inhale: Roll back onto your upper back and do a Hip-Up, using your lower Abdominal Scoop to lift the hips. Figure 5-6 shows the process of rolling onto your back. Squeeze your butt to get an extra lift.

Exhale: Returning to your Balance Point, using your Abdominal Scoop as the brake to the rolling.

Do's and don'ts

- ✔ Do think of massaging your back as you roll back and forth by using your abdominals to help you articulate each vertebra.

- ✔ Do allow your momentum to help you roll backward. Control the movement with your abdominals at the top of the Hip-Up.

- ✔ Don't allow your back to make a thumping sound, especially on the way back up. Slow down if there is any thumping, and use your abdominals to articulate into your lower back, pressing your lower back into the mat, to make a smooth movement.

- ✔ Don't roll too far back onto your neck. If you don't have a neck problem, you don't want to get one now.

Modification

Rolling Like a Ball becomes more difficult the smaller the ball you make. If you hold your hands on the front of your ankles, you tighten your ball and make it more of a control and abdominal exercise and less of a massage and articulation exercise.

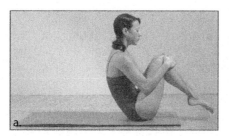
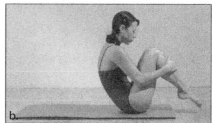
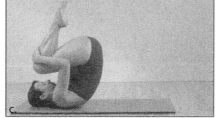

Figure 5-6:
Rolling Like
a Ball.

Single Leg Stretch

This is one of the most basic torso stability exercises in the Pilates method. Because you reach out only one leg at a time, the challenge to stability is not as demanding as it would be if you were reaching out two legs.

A torso stability exercise is one in which your torso doesn't move while your arms and/or legs are moving to challenge torso stability.

Getting set

To transition from Rolling Like a Ball, hold on to the front of your knees in a ball shape, begin to roll down your spine slowly, pushing your knees away as a counterbalance, and control the movement down to the Pilates Abdominal Position. As you roll down, pull one knee in toward your chest and straighten your other leg out to about 45 degrees from the floor (the lower the leg, the more challenging the exercise). Place your outside hand on the ankle of your bent leg, and the inside hand on the knee of your bent leg (this position maintains proper alignment of the leg). If this hand positioning is too confusing at first, simply hold the bent knee gently with both hands.

The exercise

Inhale: Switch legs 2 times on one inhale, always grabbing your bent leg with your outside hand on your ankle and your inside hand on your knee. Figure 5-7 shows the model switching legs.

Exhale: Switch legs 2 times on one exhale, grabbing on to the other bent leg with your outside hand on your ankle and your inside hand on your knee.

Repeat for 8 total breaths.

Do's and don'ts

- ✔ Do remember that this is an abdominal exercise, not a neck exercise, so you must hold the head high enough to maximize the abdominal work-out and minimize neck strain. On every exhale, think of pulling your navel in to lift up your head.

- ✔ Do keep your navel pulled in to the spine, accentuating this pulling in on every exhale.

- ✔ Don't let yourself lose the Pilates Abdominal Position by sinking down-ward; accentuate the abdominal curl up on every exhale.

- ✔ Don't continue if your neck strains. Rest your head down when your neck feels strained. Continue after a breath.

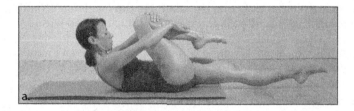

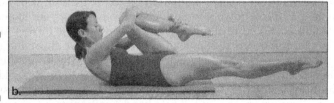

Figure 5-7:
Single Leg
Stretch.

Rising Swan

This is your first and only back extension exercise in this series (see the sidebar "The importance of being extended"). This exercise strengthens your neck, back, and butt muscles. Please include this exercise in your daily routine to counteract the negative effects of forward bending on your spine.

Getting set

Lie face down with your forehead flat on the mat, your arms bent with your elbows close to your side, and your palms facing down by your ears. Allow your legs to turn out from the top of your hip (drop your heels toward each other). You can keep a comfortable distance between the legs; if you have slim hips, you can pull your inner thighs together.

Pull your navel up off the mat so that you could slide a piece of paper under your belly and press your pubic bone down into the mat. Squeeze your butt to help press your pubic bone down. This is your powerhouse at work!

The exercise

Inhale: Maintain your position.

Exhale: Scoop your belly in, squeeze your butt, and slowly rise up from your upper back, keeping the back of your neck long and gently lifting your head off the mat (Figure 5-8a).

Pretend to see an ant on the floor below your head. Follow the ant as it crawls away from you, raising your upper back and head off the mat as it crawls up the wall in front of you.

Inhale: Hold this position, known as the Baby Swan. Test your strength by taking your hands off the mat. You don't need to be up very high to get the benefits of this exercise. Keep lifting your belly up and in toward the spine and keep squeezing your butt. Don't let your legs come off the mat!

Exhale: Return to the starting position.

Inhale: Maintain your position.

Exhale: Again scoop in your belly and squeeze your butt. Rise up a little higher this time and place your forearms down in front of you to prop you up (Figure 5-8b). You should be positioned like a sphinx. As Figure 5-9 shows, don't let your navel stay on the mat!

Inhale: Hold the sphinx position.

Exhale: Straighten your arms by pressing your hands into the mat. Protect your lower back by again pulling your belly in and squeezing your butt (Figure 5-8c). Walk your hands away if your lower back feels strained.

Inhale: Hold this position, known as the High Swan.

Exhale: Lower yourself down to the mat.

If, when in the High Swan, you feel a lot of compression or discomfort in your lower back, avoid this part of the exercise until you gain more strength in your butt and abdominals.

Finish by pushing back to the rest position. Sit on your heels with your spine rounded and relaxed forward like a fetus, as shown in Figure 5-10. See the sidebar "More on the rest position" for details.

Do's and don'ts

- ✔ Do support your head by lifting the top of your head up and away to keep your neck long and strong.
- ✔ Don't allow your lower back to sag; keep your powerhouse working overtime.

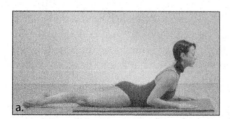
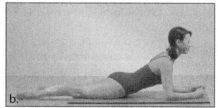

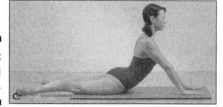

Figure 5-8:
Rising
Swan.

The importance of being extended

Whenever you lie on your belly to begin an exercise, you can be pretty sure that you'll be doing a back extension exercise. Extension exercises are ones in which you arch your back. Extension is a very important movement to practice because, if you think about it, many movements in daily life involve bending forward — which is the opposite of extension. This is because our eyes are in front of our heads, and we do everything with our arms in front of us.

Most chronic back problems are due to chronic flexion, or forward bending of the spine, and most acute spinal injuries happen in flexion. Extension exercises are a great way to counteract all that flexion that you typically do.

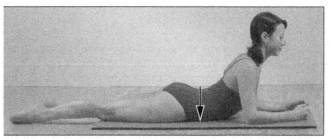

Figure 5-9:
The wrong position for Rising Swan.

Don't let your navel stay on the mat.

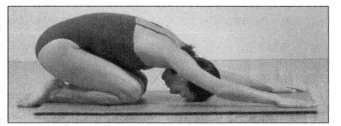

Figure 5-10:
Taking a rest in the rest position.

More on the rest position

The rest position is the best way to rest your back after doing an extension exercise (like the Rising Swan). Because you're rounded in a fetus position, your back is in a relaxed and stretched state. When in the rest position, the muscles of the back can lengthen and stretch while you just hang out and relax. Extension exercises really work the muscles of the back, which need to take a break afterward. The rest position allows for this kind of recuperation.

Roll Down

Roll Down is a beginning variation of the classic Pilates Roll Up. This exercise increases abdominal strength and articulation of the spine.

Getting set

Sit up with your knees bent and your feet flat on the floor, hip distance apart, and a comfortable distance away from your body. Extend your arms in front of you, as shown in Figure 5-11a. Think of lifting up from your lower back.

Sit up as tall as you can by imagining that you have a golden string attached to the back of the top of your head pulling you toward the sky.

The exercise

Inhale: Lift up from the base of your spine.

Exhale: Begin to roll down your spine, pulling your navel in, creating a C Curve with your lower back, and controlling the movement from the center (Figure 5-11b). Think of pressing your spine down onto the mat one vertebra at a time. Roll slowly all the way down until you're lying flat, arms by your sides (Figure 5-11c).

Inhale: Take a deep breath, expanding into your back and your lungs.

Exhale: Roll back up, thinking of lifting your head by first squeezing a tangerine under your chin, reaching your arms forward, and using the hollow abdominal muscles in a C Curve to bring you back up (Figures 5-11d and 5-11e).

Inhale: Finish the exercise by Stacking the Spine. You should end up sitting tall, in your starting position, with your arms extended in front of you and your shoulders relaxed and dropped (Figure 5-11f).

Complete 6 repetitions.

Do's and don'ts

- ✔ Do focus on using your abdominals to perform the exercise.
- ✔ Do attempt to articulate through your spine on the way down and on the way up.
- ✔ Do minimize the tension in your upper body, keeping your neck long and relaxed.
- ✔ Don't hold your breath. Use long, slow breathing to assist the movement.

Modification

If this exercise is too hard for you to do and you keep falling backward or can't get up, grab on to your legs and use your arm strength to help you control the movement down and to get yourself up.

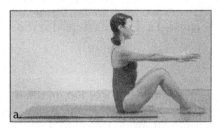

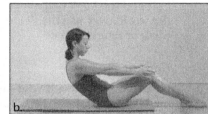

Roll down...

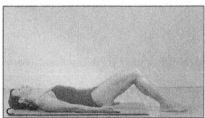

breathe in...

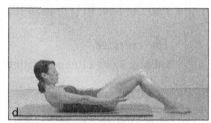

and roll back up.

Figure 5-11:
Roll Down.

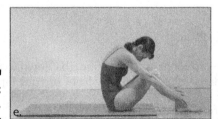

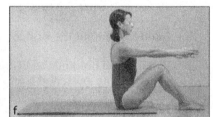

Bridge

The Bridge is an excellent torso stability exercise. When I say that an exercise is a *torso stability exercise,* that usually means that one of your goals is to keep your torso really still during the exercise. This exercise strengthens the butt and the back of the legs and teaches core stability. Physical therapists the world over use the Bridge because it's a safe exercise for those with a weak or injured back.

Getting set

Lie on your back with your knees bent and your feet flat on the floor, approximately hip distance apart. Your feet should be in a comfortable position — not too close to your butt and not too far away. You should be able to easily find the Neutral Spine. Experiment with different placements of your feet to find the best fit (Figure 5-12a).

The exercise

Inhale: Take a deep breath in, expanding into your back and your lungs.

Exhale: Keeping your torso in one flat piece, press your feet into the mat and squeeze your butt as you lift your hips up off the mat (Figure 5-12b). Come up high enough that your body makes a straight line from your shoulders to your knees. Don't press up so high that you can't see your knees (Figure 5-14 shows you what *not* to do).

Inhale: Maintain the Bridge position.

Exhale: Still holding the Bridge, think of knitting your ribs down to your belly, squeeze your butt, and try to lengthen through the front of your hips.

Inhale: Hold the Bridge position.

Exhale: Maintain Neutral Spine as you come back down to the mat.

Complete 5 repetitions.

Transition by bringing your knees into your chest to relax your back. Put one hand on each knee and slowly roll up to a sitting position.

Modification

Do the single leg variation. Place your hands on your hip bones so that you can test your hip stability. Come up to the Bridge position and, on the inhale, lift up one knee toward your chest, keeping your hips perfectly stable (Figure 5-13). Don't let your hip drop or twist as you lift up your knee. Place your foot back down on the exhale. Switch sides.

Complete 8 repetitions, alternating sides.

Do's and don'ts

- ✔ Do maintain a plank position when up in the Bridge. Try not to arch your back.

- ✔ Do maintain Neutral Spine when coming up and coming down from the Bridge.

- ✔ Do minimize the tension in your upper body, keeping your neck long and relaxed.

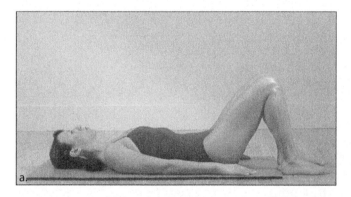

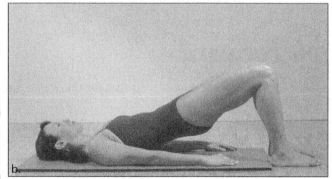

Figure 5-12: The Bridge exercise.

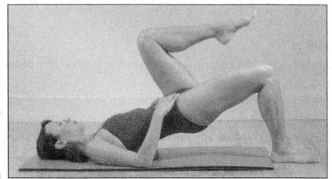

Figure 5-13: Modifying the Bridge.

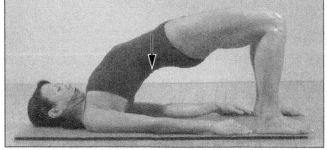

Figure 5-14: What not to do when doing the Bridge.

Don't let your back arch.

Spine Stretch Forward

Spine Stretch Forward is exactly that — a stretch for the whole spine, especially the neck and upper back.

Getting set

Sit up tall with your legs straight and spread a little wider than the width of your hips. You can bend your legs if it's impossible for you to sit up straight with your legs straight — for example, if you have tight hamstrings.

The exercise

Inhale: Sit up as tall as you can from the base of your spine. Flex your feet and reach through your heels to engage your leg muscles. Your arms should be shoulder width apart and straight ahead, with your palms facing down (Figure 5-15a).

Exhale: Round your back into a C Curve, starting by scooping out your low belly, then pulling the ribs in, and finally rounding your neck and head forward. By the end of the movement, your whole back is making a C shape, with your arms reaching forward (Figure 5-15b).

As you perform the stretch forward, imagine that you're lifting your spine up and over a barrel.

Inhale: Stack up your spine, bone by bone.

Exhale: Finish sitting tall, in your starting position, with your arms extended in front of you and your shoulders relaxed and dropped.

Complete 3 repetitions.

Do's and don'ts

- ✔ Do initiate the C Curve with your low belly.

- ✔ Don't do all the curving from your upper back; try to get your lower back rounded, too.

- ✔ Don't initiate the movement from your head; your head should trail in both parts of the exercise. When Stacking the Spine, your head is always the last thing to rise.

Modifications

Bend your knees if necessary, or sit on a small pillow if you have tight hamstrings. You can also do this exercise against a wall to practice Stacking the Spine. (Stacking the Spine is a letter of the Pilates alphabet; you can find out more in Chapter 3.)

Flexing and pointing

Flexing the foot (dorsiflexion of the ankle, foot, and toes) means pulling the toes and arch of the foot toward the calf. Your shins and your foot should make an L shape together. This action works the dorsiflexor muscles of the calves and foot. These muscles are important for proper alignment of the foot and ankle while walking.

Pointing the foot (plantarflexion of the ankle, foot, and toes) means reaching the toes and the arch of the foot away from the leg. This action strengthens the plantar flexor muscles on the back of the calf and bottom of the foot. Strong plantar flexors also assist in proper alignment when walking, help you balance when going up onto your toes, and increase power for explosive movements such as running and jumping.

When you add a pointing or flexing of the foot to an exercise, you are including the foot and calf muscles in your workout. Dancers have very strong feet and ankles because they are constantly pointing and flexing their feet, going up onto their toes and fully working their foot and calf muscles.

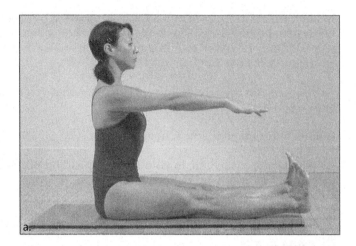

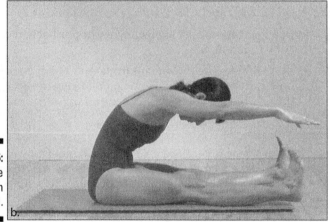

Figure 5-15:
Spine
Stretch
Forward.

Side Kicks

Side Kicks is a nice side-lying stability exercise. It focuses on control from the belly and strengthens your thighs and your butt. This exercise is not about how far you can kick your leg; it's about how stable your body can be while you move your legs freely.

Getting set

Lie on your side with your legs slightly in front of your body and slightly turned out, in the Pilates First Position. Let your head rest on your bottom hand, propped up on a bent elbow on the floor, while your top arm is bent with the palm down on the mat in front of you for stability (Figure 5-16a).

The exercise

Inhale: Flex your foot as you kick your top leg straight out in front of you, pulsing your leg once to challenge your stability (Figure 5-16b).

Exhale: Kick your leg behind you, pointing the foot, keeping it the same height as your hip, and pulsing the leg once to challenge your stability. Squeeze your butt and pull your navel in for stability.

Complete 10 repetitions on each side.

Do's and don'ts

- ✔ Do press your weight into the front palm on the floor to maintain balance throughout the exercise.
- ✔ Don't wobble like a noodle. Maintain stability in your body as your leg moves freely, especially when kicking to the back.
- ✔ Do keep your neck long and relaxed.
- ✔ Do keep your body square, shoulder over shoulder and hip over hip.

Modification

While lying on your side, instead of using one hand to support your body, put both hands behind your head and use your core strength to keep yourself stable. See Figure 5-17.

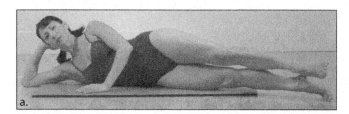

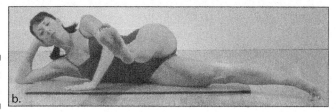

Figure 5-16: Side Kicks.

a.

b.

Figure 5-17:
The advanced hand placement for Side Kicks.

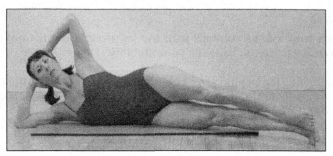

Chapter 6

Feeling Stronger Every Day: Intermediate Mat Exercises

· ·

· ·

*T*he exercises in this chapter require a certain amount of butt and gut. As you progress in the Pilates mat work, you often add more difficult exercises while doing the more basic ones as well.

I recommend starting your Pilates experience with the pre-Pilates exercises in Chapter 4 and then moving on to the beginning series in Chapter 5. If you've mastered those two series, bravo! You're ready for the intermediate series that I present in this chapter.

The intermediate series is more challenging than the previous series for a couple reasons:

✔ Because it's longer, with more exercises, it is more time consuming (you can expect to spend about twenty-five to thirty-five minutes on this series once you get familiar with it).

✔ The exercises themselves are just more difficult. They demand more from your abdominal muscles, from your coordination, and from your mind (they demand more concentration because the movements are more complex).

Pilates exercises are not meant to be done in isolation. They're meant to be done in a chain; you fluidly move from one exercise to another in a prescribed series. I present the exercises in this chapter in the order that you should do them to attain the maximum benefit.

As you progress in the Pilates series, you want to make sure that you are really flowing through the exercises. It's not enough to clunk through the exercises one by one, stopping in between. Instead, begin to try to transition seamlessly from one exercise to the next as you grow more and more independent from this book. Doing so brings a new challenge and makes your workout more aerobic.

Even though they're not officially a part of the intermediate series, try starting your workout with Coccyx Curls and Upper Abdominal Curls. Both of these exercises are described in Chapter 4, and are familiar to you if you've been doing the series in order. This is an especially good idea if you haven't warmed up at all.

The Series in This Chapter

Here's a preview of the series in this chapter. If you've been working through the series in order, from fundamental (Chapter 4) to beginning (Chapter 5) and now to intermediate, you've already mastered some of these exercises. The chapter in which I first explain them is in parentheses. The rest of the exercises are new.

- ✔ Hundred, Intermediate Level
- ✔ Roll Up
- ✔ Rolling Like a Ball (Chapter 5)
- ✔ Single Leg Stretch (Chapter 5)
- ✔ Double Leg Stretch
- ✔ Crisscross
- ✔ Scissors
- ✔ Open Leg Rocker
- ✔ Single Leg Kick
- ✔ Double Leg Kick
- ✔ Side Kicks (Chapter 5 and Chapter 9 for more variations)
- ✔ Teaser, Modified
- ✔ The Seal

Hundred, Intermediate Level

This exercise is excellent for increasing torso stability and abdominal strength, but you may find it difficult to keep your head up for the hundred counts that give this exercise its name. Never continue if your neck feels strained; see the "Do's and don'ts" section for ways to protect your neck. As you get stronger in your neck and your abdominals, you will not notice this strain.

This increases the difficulty of the exercise because the weight of the legs puts a little more load on the torso, forcing the abdominals to work a little harder. In the intermediate Hundred, your legs are straight. In the beginning version of the Hundred, your knees are bent in the tabletop position.

This exercise calls for accordion and percussive breathing. For accordion breathing, imagine that your rib cage is an accordion. On the inhale the accordion expands laterally, and on the exhale the accordion squeezes back together. Percussive breathing is forced exhalation using the abdominal muscles; think of forcing the air out in short percussive blows.

Getting set

Lie on your back with your knees bent and feet up in the air. Your knees and hips should be in the tabletop position, inner thighs squeezing together, knees bent at a 90-degree angle, arms down by your sides.

The exercise

Inhale: Reach your arms straight up with your palms facing forward, as shown in Figure 6-1a.

Exhale: As you reach your arms back down to the floor, lift your head and roll up to the Pilates Abdominal Position with the shoulder blades just off the mat (for details on the Pilates Abdominal Position, see the Pilates alphabet in Chapter 3). Simultaneously straighten your legs up to the sky, as shown in Figure 6-1b.

Why do I say *reach* your arms down to the floor instead of *lower* them down? To remind you to keep your arms stretched and long as you drop them.

As you roll up into your Pilates Abdominal Position, think of squeezing a tangerine under your chin. This image helps you keep space between your chin and your chest so that your neck isn't overstretched.

Keep your legs in the Pilates First Position (a letter of the Pilates alphabet, described in Chapter 3), slightly turned out from the hip, with your inner thighs pulling together. Your palms gently slap the floor in a quick, percussive rhythm.

Inhale: Inhale deeply for 5 beats (keep the rhythm with your arms), using accordion breathing.

Exhale: Using percussive breathing, exhale for 5 beats (saying "shh, shh, shh, shh, shh").

Hold the position and continue pulsing your arms for 10 breaths, which is 100 total beats (5 for each inhale and 5 for each exhale).

Lower your head to the mat and bring your knees into your chest to relax your back. Then extend your arms and legs long on the mat to get ready for the Roll Up.

Do's and don'ts

- ✔ Do remember that this is an abdominal exercise, not a neck exercise. You must keep your head high enough to maximize the abdominal workout and minimize neck strain.

- ✔ Do press your lower back into the mat by using your Abdominal Scoop, especially on the exhale.

- ✔ Do think of reaching long away from you with your fingers and try to think of pulsing your arms from your back, imagining that the movement of the arms initiates at the shoulder blades.

- ✔ Don't continue in this position if your neck strains. Put one hand behind your head to support the neck; switch hands at 50 beats.

- ✔ Don't let yourself lose the Pilates Abdominal Position by sinking downward; accentuate the abdominal curl on every exhale.

Modification

To make the Hundred more advanced, lower your legs to a 45-degree angle, making sure to keep your lower back flat on the mat by scooping your abs and squeezing your butt.

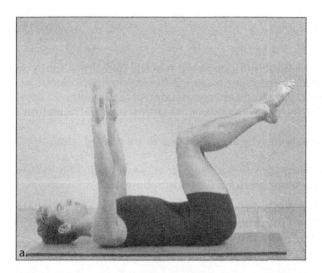

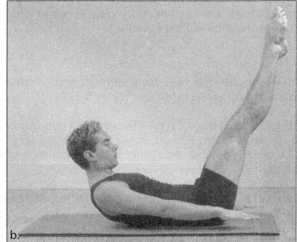

Figure 6-1:
The
intermediate
level
Hundred.

Roll Up

The Roll Up is the more difficult version of the Roll Down that you do in the beginning series I present in Chapter 5. Before doing this exercise, you should be able to do a Roll Down with control and mastery. Like the Roll Down, the Roll Up increases abdominal strength and articulation of the spine.

There are two reasons why the Roll Up is more difficult than the Roll Down:

- ✔ You begin with your legs straight instead of bent. This makes your abdominals work harder to get you rolling up.
- ✔ In the Roll Down, your arms stay by your sides, whereas in the Roll Up your arms are reaching upward as you come off the mat. This also puts more load on your abdominals.

Getting set

Lie down on your back with arms extended by your ears and your legs straight on the floor in the Pilates First Position.

The exercise

Inhale: Breathe in deeply. Stretch your arms and legs away from each other like you do when waking up in the morning (Figure 6-2a).

Exhale: Lift your arms up to the sky, palms forward. As your arms become perpendicular to the floor, lift your head, squeezing an imaginary tangerine under your chin. Squeeze your butt and inner thighs together and scoop your abdominals to initiate the rolling up movement (Figure 6-2b).

Inhale: Stretch forward over your legs as you pull your navel in, hollowing your belly in opposition to the forward stretch (Figure 6-2c).

Exhale: Initiate the Roll Down by squeezing your butt and inner thighs together and begin to roll down your spine, creating a C Curve with your back. Control the movement from the center by pulling your navel in toward your spine (Figure 6-2d). Think of pressing your spine down onto the mat one vertebra at a time. Roll slowly all the way down to lying flat, your arms reaching above your ears, and begin again.

Complete 6 repetitions. Finish the last one by lying flat on your back with your arms down by your sides. Bend your knees and bring them up to your chest, grabbing onto them with your hands. Roll yourself up to sitting to prepare for Rolling Like a Ball.

Do's and don'ts

- ✔ Do focus on using your abdominals to perform the exercise.

- ✔ Do attempt to articulate through your spine on the way down and on the way up.

- ✔ Do minimize the tension in your upper body; keep your neck long and relaxed.

- ✔ Don't let your feet or legs lift off the floor as you roll up.

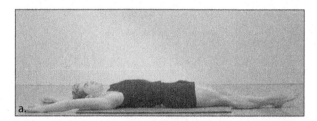

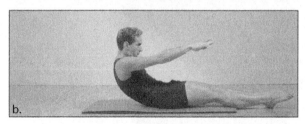

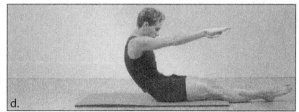

After stretching forward...

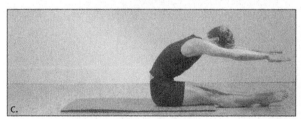

Figure 6-2:
Roll Up.

control the movement back down.

Rolling Like a Ball

At this point in the series, do the Rolling Like a Ball exercise that I introduce in the beginning series. See Chapter 5 for instructions and Figure 6-3 for photos. Complete 6 repetitions and then slowly roll down to your Pilates Abdominal Position, allowing one knee to bend into your chest (outside hand on the ankle, inside hand on the knee) and straightening the other leg as you transition into the Single Leg Stretch.

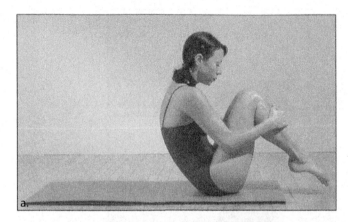

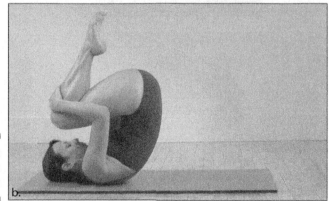

Figure 6-3:
Rolling Like
a Ball.

Single Leg Stretch

After Rolling Like a Ball, do the Single Leg Stretch. See Chapter 5 for instructions and Figure 6-4 for photos. Complete 20 repetitions, alternating sides. Transition to the Double Leg Stretch by bringing both knees into your chest, holding one knee with each hand.

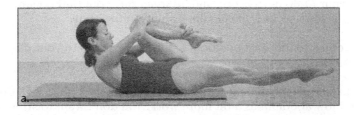

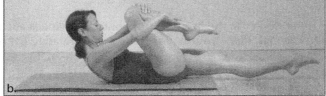

Figure 6-4:
Single Leg
Stretch.

Double Leg Stretch

The Double Leg Stretch is much more challenging than the Single Leg Stretch. Not only are you supporting two legs rather than one, but your arms are also added to the equation, making torso stability that much more difficult. This exercise requires a huge amount of abdominal strength and requires full-torso stability, meaning both upper and lower torso stability.

A torso stability exercise is one in which your torso does not move while your arms and/or legs are moving to challenge this stability.

As you perform this exercise, you should reach your legs only as low as you can while still maintaining absolute stability in your torso. Absolute stability means that your back should not arch off the mat at all and the belly must stay pulled in and scooped. If you feel any discomfort in your lower back, you are dropping your legs too low, meaning your abdominal muscles can't support their weight. This may cause injury to the back, so please bring your legs back up!

Getting set

Lie on your back with your knees on your chest, holding onto one knee with each hand. Roll up into the Pilates Abdominal Position (Figure 6-5a).

The exercise

Inhale: Send your arms and legs out into a V, your arms by your ears and your legs at a 45-degree angle to the floor. Keep your lower back in contact with the mat with your Abdominal Scoop and by squeezing your butt (Figure 6-5b). Hold this position for a second, feeling the stability in the body.

Exhale: Return to the start position, pulling your knees to your chest and hollowing your belly.

You can finish this movement with a baby Hip-Up (see Chapter 4). Doing so gives your low abdominals a bit more work. You don't want to stress the Hip-Up too much; hence, a "baby" Hip-Up.

Complete 6 repetitions. On the last one, hold onto your knees and lower your head down to the mat. Place your hands behind your head to get ready for Crisscross.

Do's and don'ts

- ✔ Do keep your belly scooped in when your limbs are extended.

- ✔ Don't let yourself lose the Pilates Abdominal Position by sinking downward. People tend to let the head drop back when their arms are extended by their ears. To counteract this tendency, keep your focus on your belly the whole time.

- ✔ Don't continue if your neck strains. Bring your head back down to the mat. Continue after a breath.

- ✔ Don't continue if your lower back strains. Modify the exercise by reaching your legs straight up to the sky until you gain more abdominal strength.

Modification

The lower your legs, the more abdominal work is needed to keep your lower back flat on the mat. Lower your legs as low as you can while still maintaining contact with the mat with your lower back.

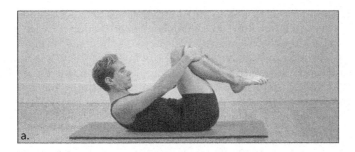

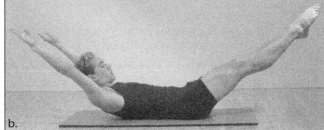

Figure 6-5:
Double Leg
Stretch.

Crisscross

Crisscross is similar to the Single Leg Stretch, but it adds a twist to the body that strengthens the oblique abdominal muscles. If this exercise is too difficult for you, repeat the Single Leg Stretch from earlier in the series instead.

Getting set

Bring your hands behind your head and roll up into the Pilates Abdominal Position with your knees bent and in the air.

The exercise

Inhale: Reach one elbow to the opposite knee and extend your other leg long in front of you. Then alternate sides, reaching your other elbow to your other knee. Imagine pulling your shoulder blade off the mat and twisting from your back muscles as you twist your body. Do not drop out of the Pilates Abdominal Position; try to keep your shoulder blades off the mat. Figure 6-6 shows the crisscrossing motion.

Exhale: Continue the crisscrossing motion, making 2 twists on the exhale.

Do 2 movements for each inhale and 2 movements for each exhale. Repeat for 8 total breaths (an inhale and an exhale is a breath). Finish by bringing your knees into your chest and lowering your head to the mat. Straighten out your legs and split them apart, leaving one on the mat and the other pointing up to the sky. Grab onto the leg that's pointing up, as high on the leg as you can reach, while rolling up to the Pilates Abdominal Position. This gets you set for Scissors.

Do's and don'ts

✔ Do keep your navel pulled into your spine, accentuating this pulling in on every exhale.

✔ Do keep your elbows wide and make sure you're twisting from your torso; move your torso, not just your elbows.

✔ Don't let yourself lose the Pilates Abdominal Position by sinking downward; think of rotating the body without touching your shoulder blades to the mat.

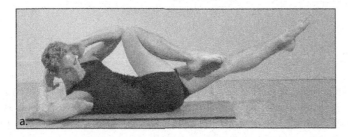

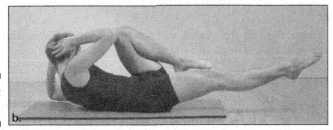

Figure 6-6: Crisscross.

Scissors

Scissors is both an abdominal exercise and a hamstring stretch. If straightening your leg to a 90-degree angle is difficult, then you may want to start by stretching out the hamstring first and then proceed to this exercise. See Figure 6-7 for a hamstring stretch.

Getting set

Start from the hamstring stretch position, holding onto one leg with the other leg straight on the floor. Roll up into the Pilates Abdominal Position.

The exercise

Inhale: Extend one leg to the sky and grab it below the ankle. If you have tight hamstrings, simply hold your leg closer to your knee and allow the knee to bend a little. Straighten your other leg in front of you, keeping it slightly above the mat (Figure 6-8a).

Exhale: Switch legs, and as you pull the other leg toward your body pull it two times quickly to make a double pulsing motion (Figure 6-8b).

Complete 10 breath cycles, or 20 total leg pulls.

VISUALIZE

"Nose to your knee and knee to your nose." Always think of raising your head a little higher to touch your nose to your knees. Doing so will keep your abs working!

Do's and don'ts

- ✔ Do keep your navel pulled into the spine, accentuating the scoop on every exhale.

- ✔ Do keep your legs as straight as possible.

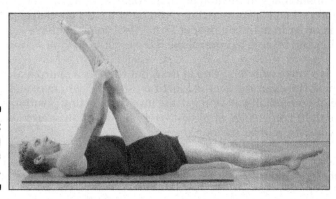

Figure 6-7:
Stretching
the
hamstring.

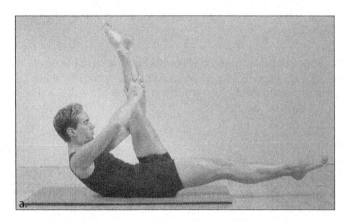

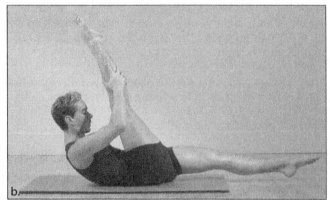

Figure 6-8:
Scissors.

Open Leg Rocker

This is the second of three rolling exercises in the Pilates mat series. Open Leg Rocker is substantially more difficult than Rolling Like a Ball, versions of which are in Chapters 4 and 5. For one thing, you must have a good deal of hamstring flexibility in order to maintain proper form. Also, you must have a good deal of coordination and be able to control the movement from your center.

This exercise may seem daunting at first, but there is a sharp learning curve as you repeat the exercise. By the fourth or fifth roll, you may feel a little more sure of yourself. If you find getting into the starting position difficult because of tight hamstrings or a tight back, simply allow your knees to bend and hold your legs closer to your knees.

You may want to do Spine Stretch Forword before doing the Open Leg Rocker. See the sidebar "Making the intermediate series longer" for more information.

As when doing any rolling exercise, be careful not to roll onto your neck!

Getting set

Start by sitting up in the Balance Point, with your knees bent and open to the sides, feet off the floor, and your hands holding the outsides of your ankles.

To practice finding your balance, first straighten one leg out to the side in front of you, maintaining your Balance Point position and deep Abdominal Scoop. Bend your knee back in and then repeat with your other leg. Figures 6-9a and 6-9b show you how to find your balance.

Now to find the starting position, extend both legs at the same time into a V shape in front of you. Keep your low belly hollowed and remain in your Balance Point position, balanced just behind your tailbone to feel your belly helping you balance. Figure 6-9c shows the starting position.

The exercise

Inhale: Roll onto your upper back and do a Hip-Up (Figure 6-9d). Use your lower Abdominal Scoop to lift your hips, and squeeze your butt to get an extra lift.

Exhale: Return to your Balance Point, using your Abdominal Scoop as a brake to halt the rolling motion.

Complete 6 repetitions.

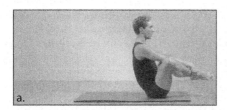
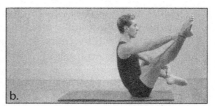
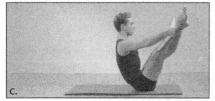
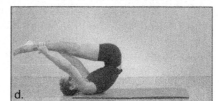

Figure 6-9:
Open Leg
Rocker.

Making the intermediate series longer

If you're ready for even more of a challenge, try adding Spine Stretch Forward (from Chapter 5) and the Bridge (also from Chapter 5) to the intermediate series. As the series gets longer, you get even more of a workout, and these exercises are ideal add-ons. I like to do Spine Stretch Forward after doing Scissors and the Bridge after doing Open Leg Rocker, but you can experiment.

Do's and don'ts

✔ Do think of massaging your back by using your Abdominal Scoop to help you articulate each vertebra.

✔ Do allow your momentum to help you roll backward, and control the movement with your abdominals at the top of the Hip-Up.

✔ Don't allow your back to make a thumping sound, especially on the way back up. Use your Abdominal Scoop to help you articulate the rolling — especially through your lower back — to make a smooth movement.

Single Leg Kick

My boyfriend giggled when he saw me doing this exercise. Yes, there is something a little silly about the look of this one, but it's a great exercise. It strengthens your back muscles, trains your shoulders to drop down the back, and simultaneously stretches the front of your legs and hips (the quadriceps muscles) while toning the back of your thighs (the hamstrings) and your butt (the gluteus muscles).

Getting set

Start by lying on your belly, and then prop yourself up like a sphinx on your elbows. Figure 6-10a shows the proper position, but it's a little more complicated than the photo may indicate:

✔ Your forearms should be shoulder width apart, with your hands in fists pressing into the mat.

✔ Your legs are parallel, hip distance apart, your navel is up off the mat, and your pubic bone is pressed down into the mat. Squeeze your butt to accomplish this tucking under of your pelvis. This is your powerhouse at work!

> ✔ Your elbows are pushed into the mat while your shoulder blades are pulled down your back. Really try to feel the muscles underneath your shoulder blades pulling and maintaining this shoulder position while you do the exercise.

The exercise

Breathing continuously: Kick your right heel to your butt with a double beat, the first beat with a pointed foot and the second beat with a flexed foot (Figures 6-10b and 6-10c). Point your foot as you straighten your leg to the mat. Alternate legs.

Complete 10 repetitions on each leg, or 20 total movements. Finish by coming back down onto your belly, bringing your head to one side, and allowing your hands to interlace behind your back. Now you're ready to flow into the Double Leg Kick.

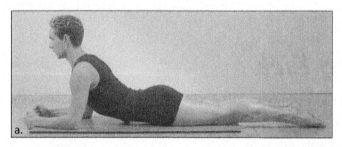

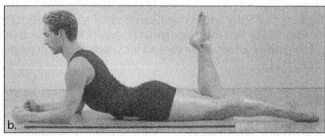

Pointed foot

Figure 6-10:
Single Leg
Kick.

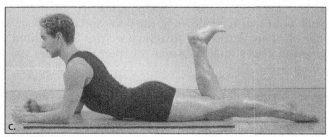

Flexed foot

If you feel yourself sinking in the middle and your lower back compressing, recharge your powerhouse by finding your Abdominal Scoop and squeezing your butt anew. If your lower back continues to hurt, stop and push back to the rest position (sitting on your heels in a fetus position, with your back rounded and head and neck relaxed forward, your arms outstretched in front of you).

Do's and don'ts

✔ Do maintain a lifted upper body and absolute stability in your torso during this exercise.

✔ Do support your head by lifting the top of your head up and away to keep your neck long and strong.

✔ Do keep pressing your elbows into the mat to keep your shoulders pulling down your back.

✔ Do keep your inner thighs and knees glued together.

✔ Don't allow your back to sag; keep your powerhouse working overtime.

Double Leg Kick

This exercise opens your chest, strengthens your back, and tones the back of your legs and your buttocks.

Getting set

Start by lying on your belly with your head turned to one side. Bend your arms behind your back and interlace your fingers. Place your hands as high on your back as you comfortably can and let your elbows drop down onto the mat (Figure 6-11a).

The exercise

Inhale: Kick both heels to your butt, making three beats. Be sure to not let your back arch when doing this movement; squeeze your butt to counteract this tendency (Figure 6-11b).

Exhale: Extend your legs back down to the floor and reach your arms back as you arch your back up off the mat. Reach your arms long behind you and think of squeezing your shoulder blades together to increase the stretch in your chest (Figure 6-11c).

Inhale: Return to lying flat, turning your head in the opposite direction and again kicking your heels.

Complete 4 repetitions and press back to the rest position. Sit on your heels in a fetus position, with your back rounded forward and your arms on the floor in front of you (Figure 6-12). After you've rested your back for a few breaths, roll onto your side for Side Kicks.

Do's and don'ts

- ✔ Do keep your Abdominal Scoop throughout the exercise.

- ✔ Don't allow your head to sink back into your shoulders. Instead, lengthen the back of your neck.

- ✔ Don't allow your back to sag; keep your powerhouse working overtime.

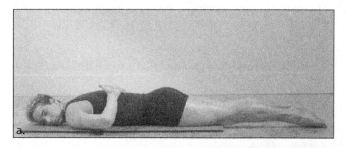

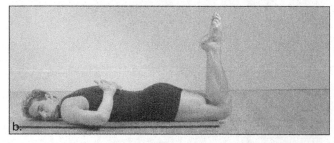

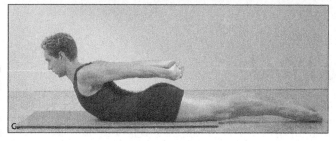

Figure 6-11: Double Leg Kick.

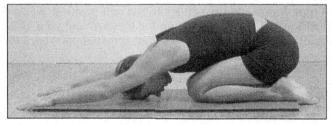

Figure 6-12:
Ahhh . . . the
rest
position.

Side Kicks

After you've been in the rest position, roll over to your side and do Side Kicks. For instructions, see Chapter 5. For photos, see Figure 6-13. Complete 10 repetitions.

For Side Kick variations that give you more of a workout, see Chapter 9.

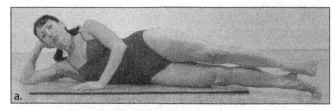

a.

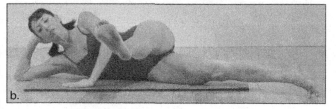

Figure 6-13:
Side Kicks.

b.

Teaser, Modified

I have no idea why this exercise is called Teaser. Maybe because you tease your abdominals into working? Whatever! Anyway, the Teasers are some of the most difficult of all the abdominal exercises in the Pilates method. By having your legs suspended in the air, you are forced to use your deep abdominal muscles.

This exercise requires balance, center strength, and a sense of humor. Like the Balance Point exercise, the Teaser is one of the best I know to find your deep abdominal muscles. You cannot cheat and use only your hip flexors (the muscles that lift up your legs) in this exercise, which is often the case with abdominal exercises. The Balance Point is the seed of all the Teaser exercises, so if this movement feels too advanced, go back to the Balance Point exercise in Chapter 4 for a while.

Getting set

Come up to the Balance Point position — you should be sitting up, knees bent and feet off the floor, holding the back of your thighs with your hands (wrapping your hands around the outside of the legs). You should be balanced right behind your tailbone (coccyx), with your lower back rounded and your belly hollowed out.

The exercise

Inhale: Release your arms and let them reach gently up in front of you, trying not to come out of your Balance Point position (Figure 6-14a). You should feel your Abdominal Scoop working now to keep your balance.

Exhale: Begin to roll down your spine, keeping your legs up in a tabletop position, squeezing them together with the calves parallel to the floor (Figure 6-14b). Pull your navel in and control the movement from the center. Control the movement down until you're lying on the mat. Allow your arms to trail you as you lie down, bringing them down by your sides with your palms facing up.

Inhale: Take a deep breath in, expanding into your back and lungs.

Exhale: Initiate the roll up by feeling the shoulder blades pulling down your back as you reach your arms forward and roll back up to the Balance Point position.

Complete 6 repetitions. On the last one finish up in your Balance Point. Bringing your feet back down to the mat, open your knees and grab around the outside of your ankles to get set for the final exercise, The Seal!

If you're having difficulty controlling the rolling down and up, cheat by grabbing onto your thighs to allow your arms to help you complete the movement.

Do's and don'ts

- ✔ Do focus on using your abdominals to perform the exercise.
- ✔ Do attempt to articulate through your spine on the way down and on the way up.

✔ Do minimize the tension in your upper body; keep your neck long and relaxed.

✔ Don't allow your legs to move out and in, but keep them as still as possible in the tabletop position.

✔ Don't continue if you can't control your movements. Instead, go back to the Balance Point exercise.

Modification

To make this exercise easier, try starting it with one foot on the mat and the other up in the tabletop position. This position will give you more control as you roll up and down your spine. When you've got this down, try the exercise with both legs up!

If you want a more difficult variation, try doing the same exact exercise, except keep your legs straight (without any bend at the knee). Have your legs at a 45-degree angle to the floor.

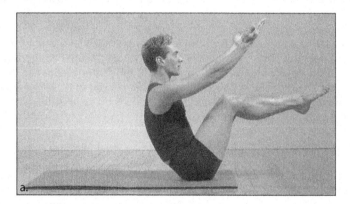

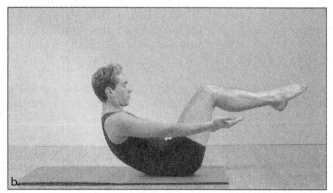

Figure 6-14:
A modified version of Teaser.

The Fives: Five abdominal exercises to do every day

If you want ten minutes of excruciating ab work, the Fives are for you. These exercises, when done regularly, keep your middle taut and prevent injury to the back. You can also use the Fives as a warm-up for doing other exercise forms, because these exercises will awaken your middle and help your form, no matter what you choose to do with your body.

Remember, don't push yourself if you aren't ready for these exercises. If you feel your lower back straining, please modify the exercises by raising your legs higher off the floor. The lower you reach your legs, the more work your abdominal muscles have to do to stabilize the spine. So please be aware of your level; the thing to watch out for is what I call "pooching." If you see your belly protrude suddenly when you reach your legs out for one of these exercises, you need to modify by lifting up the legs.

I like to insert Rolling Like a Ball into this series to break up the burn and to give the back a little rest after the Hundred. So you could call these exercises the Sixes, but it just doesn't sound as good.

- ✔ Hundred (Chapter 5, 6, or 7 — variations are in each of these chapters)
- ✔ Rolling Like a Ball (Chapter 5)
- ✔ Single Leg Stretch (Chapter 5)
- ✔ Crisscross (Chapter 6)
- ✔ Double Leg Stretch (Chapter 6)
- ✔ Scissors (Chapter 6)

The Seal

I think The Seal was developed to promote humility. This exercise often concludes a mat class, and it lets students leave class with a smile. Yes, it is a silly-looking exercise, but I love it for teaching the concept of Levitation. Levitation is a more advanced Pilates concept that combines a Hip-Up with a buttocks lift.

As when performing any rolling exercise, do not roll onto your neck.

Getting set

Start by sitting up in the Balance Point position, balanced slightly behind your tailbone with your knees bent and open to the sides, your feet together and slightly off the floor, and your hands grabbing your ankles from the inside (Figure 6-15a).

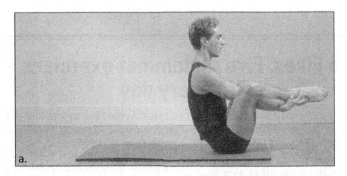

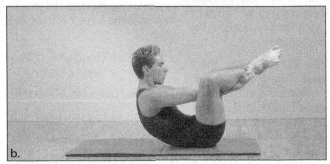

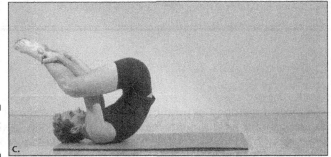

Figure 6-15:
The Seal.

The exercise

Inhale: Clap the soles of your feet together 3 times (like a seal), roll back onto your upper back, and do a Hip-Up (Figure 6-15b shows the model rolling back). Use your lower Abdominal Scoop to lift the hips and squeeze your butt to get an extra lift. Clap your feet again 3 times at your highest point (Figure 6-15c).

Exhale: Return to your Balance Point, using your Abdominal Scoop as the brake to the momentum. Again, clap your feet 3 times.

Complete 6 repetitions . . . and you're done with the intermediate series! Congrats.

Do's and don'ts

- ✔ Do think of massaging your back using your abdominals to help you articulate each vertebra.

- ✔ Do allow your momentum to help you roll backward, and control the movement with your abdominals at the top of the Hip-Up.

- ✔ Don't allow your back to make a thumping sound, especially on the way back up. Use your abdominals to pull into your lower back to make a smooth movement.

- ✔ Don't roll too far back onto your neck. Even if you don't have neck problems, you don't want to start having them now.

Modification

The hardest part of this exercise is maintaining the Levitation or Hip-Up position long enough to clap 3 times. So instead, start with one clap on your way back and then add another and another as you gain control.

Chapter 7

More Than a Washboard: The Advanced Mat Series

Don't try the advanced series until you can complete the intermediate series in Chapter 6 with confidence and ease. You need core strength and core stability before you can move on to the advanced exercises. Once you've built up your core, you'll be able to add on the fancy variations that make up the advanced work.

Not only are the exercises more challenging in the advanced series, but the workout gets a lot longer, as you may notice. So part of becoming more advanced is gaining endurance as well as strength — a powerful combination!

I think it's a good idea to warm up with Coccyx Curls and Upper Abdominal Curls before launching into this series, especially if you're not warmed up at all. Both of these exercises are described in full in Chapter 4.

The Series in This Chapter

Get ready for the hard stuff. The advanced series includes all the exercises in the following list. If you've done the exercises in the previous chapter, you've already done quite a few of these exercises. I include chapter references for those exercises that aren't new.

✔ Hundred, Advanced Version

✔ Roll Up (Chapter 6)

✔ Rollover

- Rolling Like a Ball (Chapter 5)
- Single Leg Stretch (Chapter 5)
- Double Leg Stretch (Chapter 6)
- Crisscross (Chapter 6)
- Scissors (Chapter 6)
- Spine Stretch Forward (Chapter 5)
- Open Leg Rocker (Chapter 6)
- Corkscrew
- Rising Swan (Chapter 5)
- The Saw
- Single Leg Kick (Chapter 6)
- Double Leg Kick (Chapter 6)
- Neck Pull
- Shoulder Bridge
- Spine Twist
- The Jackknife
- Side Kicks (Chapter 5)
- Teaser, Advanced Version
- Hip Flexor Stretch
- Hip Circles
- Swimming
- Control Front
- Kneeling Side Kicks
- Side Bend/Advanced Mermaid
- The Seal (Chapter 6)
- Pilates Push-Up

Hundred, Advanced Version

This exercise is excellent for developing torso stability and abdominal strength. In the advanced version of this exercise, your legs are straight and dropped to at least a 45-degree angle. In order to keep absolute stability in your torso with the weight of your legs dropping down, the abdominals need to work much harder than in the intermediate version (with the legs straight up) or in the beginning version (with the knees bent).

Getting set

Lie on your back with your legs in the tabletop position (your hips and knees bent at 90-degree angles and your inner thighs squeezing together) and your arms by your sides.

The exercise

Inhale: Reach your arms up to the sky, palms facing forward (Figure 7-1a).

Exhale: As you reach your arms back down to the floor, lift your head and roll up to the Pilates Abdominal Position, with your shoulder blades just off the mat. Simultaneously, straighten your legs, stretching them forward in front of you at about a 45-degree angle to the ground. Figure 7-1b shows this position.

Lower your legs only as far as you can while maintaining a scooped-out belly and flattened lower back. Keep your legs in the Pilates First Position (see Chapter 3), slightly turned out from your hips, your knees facing away from each other, and your inner thighs pulling together. Gently slap your palms on the floor in a quick, percussive rhythm.

Inhale: Pump your arms up and down for 5 beats, making very small pulses.

Exhale: Keep the rhythm by pumping your arms up and down for 5 more beats. (Say, "Shh, shh, shh, shh, shh.")

Hold this position and continue the arm pulsing for 10 full breaths (10 beats per breath makes 100 total beats).

If your neck feels strained, put one hand behind your head to support your neck, and switch hands at 50 beats.

Relax your head down to the mat, bring your knees into your chest, and gently circle your knees to relax your back. Rest for 1 or more breaths before continuing in the series. This exercise really works your abdominals and neck muscles, so you may need to rest your head on the mat for a moment before continuing. Once you're ready to move on, lengthen your legs out in front of you and reach your arms above your head to get ready for the Roll Up.

Do's and don'ts

✔ Do remember that this is primarily an abdominal exercise, not a neck exercise. You must maintain the head high enough to maximize the abdominal workout and minimize neck strain.

✔ Do press your lower back into the mat by using your Abdominal Scoop, and squeeze your butt to help stabilize your lower back.

✔ Do think of reaching long away from yourself with your fingers and try to think of pumping your arms from the back.

✔ Do think of squeezing a tangerine under your chin to keep a little space between your chin and your chest so that you don't overstretch the back of your neck.

✔ Don't let yourself lose the Pilates Abdominal Position by sinking downward; accentuate the abdominal curl up on every exhale.

Modification

To make the Hundred easier, raise your legs straight up to the sky as you pulse your arms. This is the intermediate version presented in Chapter 6.

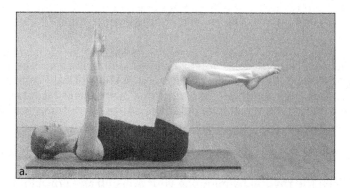

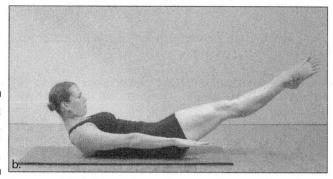

Figure 7-1: Hundred, Advanced Version.

Roll Up

After doing the Hundred, do the Roll Up. Complete 5 repetitions. Chapter 6 contains a full description. If you've done the series in Chapter 6, Figure 7-2 can refresh your memory. Finish by rolling down to your back, your arms down by your sides, and bend your knees and lift them straight up to the sky to get ready for the Rollover.

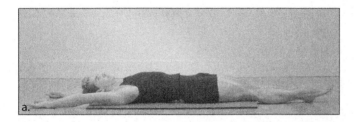

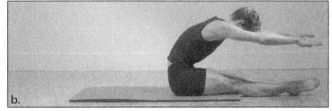

Figure 7-2:
Roll Up.

Rollover

The Rollover demands a great amount of core strength. When you do it right, it teaches spinal articulation, and it's a delicious stretch for your back and neck muscles. If you have problems getting your hips up and over your head (if you have a heavy bottom or tight lower back), then you may have problems with this exercise. Go back to the Hip-Up (Chapter 4) and practice that instead.

If you have lower back or neck problems, avoid this exercise.

Getting set

Lie flat on your back with your arms down by your sides, your palms facing downward, your legs straight up to the sky and slightly turned out from the top of the hips, and your knees facing away from each other. Squeeze your inner thighs and heels together in the Pilates First Position (Figure 7-3a).

The exercise

Inhale: Take a deep breath in.

Exhale: Squeeze your butt, pull your belly in, and lift your legs up and over your head. As shown in Figure 7-3b, your legs should stop once they're parallel to the floor; don't let your toes touch the floor behind you. Don't roll onto your neck, but stop and balance on your shoulders instead.

Inhale: Open your legs to hip distance apart as you begin to slowly roll back down your spine (Figure 7-3c). Flex your feet and think of reaching your heels long toward the wall behind you.

Exhale: Continue rolling down your spine, pressing your palms and arms into the floor to control the movement. Allow your legs to drop back down toward the floor in front of you, but only as low as you can while still maintaining a flattened lower back (Figure 7-3d). Use your Abdominal Scoop and your butt squeeze to help keep your lower back flat on the mat. Don't let your lower back arch off the mat even a little!

Inhale: Squeeze your legs together and begin the sequence again.

Complete 3 repetitions. Then reverse the leg position by starting the exercise with your legs open, and squeeze them together at the top of the Rollover. Complete 3 repetitions of this variation.

End by bending your knees into your chest and gently circle your knees to help release your lower back. Get ready for Rolling Like a Ball by holding on to both knees and rolling up to a sitting position (the Balance Point).

Do's and don'ts

✔ Do keep the movement flowing and controlled.

✔ Don't roll up onto your neck. Think of keeping your neck long.

Modifications

To make this exercise easier, when you return from the Rollover, bring your legs back to this 90-degree angle and begin to practice lowering your legs little by little every time you repeat the exercise. Lower your legs as low as you can while still keeping your lower back flat on the mat. If your lower back arches off *at all* as you lower your legs, stop and bring your legs back up again. Doing so protects your lower back. As you gain more abdominal strength, you'll be able to lower your legs quite close to the floor and still maintain a stable torso.

If your back is tight and you'd like to get more stretch out of this exercise, start the first Rollover and stop at the top, with your legs overhead, and grab on to each calf with your hands. Roll slowly down your spine, using your arms to help you stretch into your back. Then continue with the sequence.

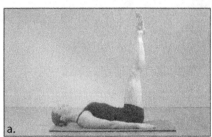
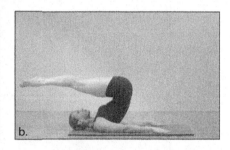

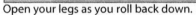
Open your legs as you roll back down.

Figure 7-3: Rollover.

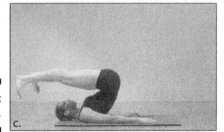
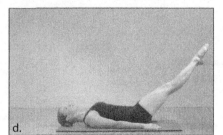

Rolling Like a Ball

At this point in the series, do the Rolling Like a Ball exercise that I introduce in the beginning series. Refer to Chapter 5 for complete instructions on how to do this exercise, shown here in Figure 7-4. Complete 6 repetitions and then slowly roll down into your Pilates Abdominal Position, allowing one knee to bend into your chest (with your outside hand on the ankle and your inside hand on the knee) and straightening the other leg as you transition into the Single Leg Stretch.

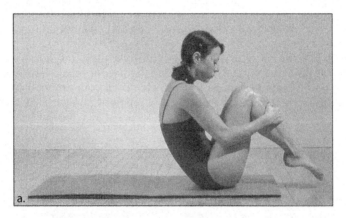

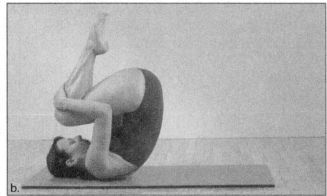

Figure 7-4:
Rolling Like
a Ball.

Single Leg Stretch

You can turn to Chapter 5 for detailed instructions for the Single Leg Stretch, shown here in Figure 7-5. Complete 20 repetitions, alternating sides. Finish by bringing both knees into your chest, holding one knee with each hand, and rest your head back on the mat to transition to the Double Leg Stretch.

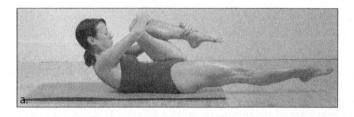

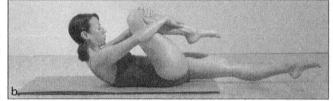

Figure 7-5:
Single Leg
Stretch.

Double Leg Stretch

The Double Leg Stretch is described in detail in Chapter 6. Figure 7-6 can help you remember how it's done. Complete 6 repetitions. On the last one, hold on to your knees and lower your head down to the mat. Place your hands behind your head to get ready for Crisscross.

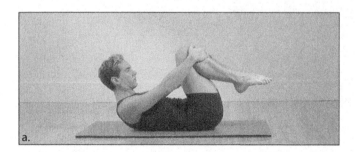

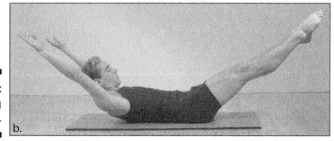

Figure 7-6:
Double Leg
Stretch.

Crisscross

You can find this exercise in Chapter 6, and Figure 7-7 shows how it's done. Complete 20 repetitions, alternating sides, and finish by bringing your knees into your chest and lowering your head to the mat. Straighten out your legs, but leave one on the mat and hold the other up to the sky, grabbing on to it as high as you can while rolling up to the Pilates Abdominal Position. This position gets you set for the Scissors.

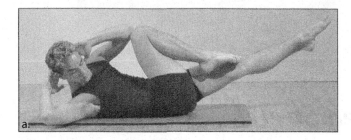

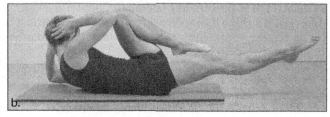

Figure 7-7:
Crisscross.

Scissors

The Scissors exercise, from Chapter 6, comes next. See Figure 7-8, but remember that you can start with a basic hamstring stretch, if you need to. Repeat for 20 leg pulls. Bring both knees into your chest and, grabbing on to them, roll up to sitting and straighten your legs out in front of you, a little wider than hip distance apart, to get ready for Spine Stretch Forward.

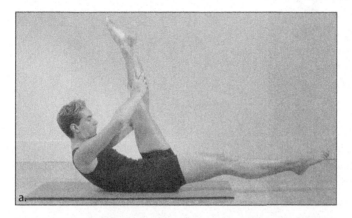

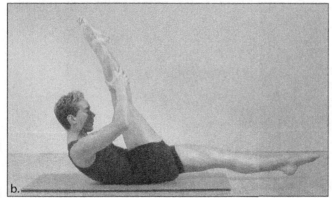

Figure 7-8:
Scissors.

Spine Stretch Forward

At this point in the series, give your back a good stretch. Spine Stretch Forward is described in Chapter 5 and shown in Figure 7-9. Do 3 times.

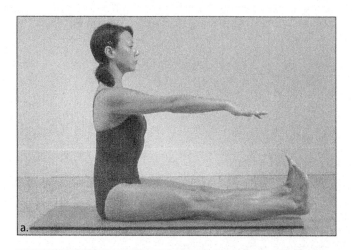

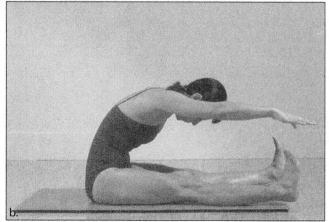

Figure 7-9:
Spine
Stretch
Forward.

Open Leg Rocker

Open Leg Rocker is described in Chapter 6. Figure 7-10 shows you how to perform it. Complete 6 repetitions and finish by bending your knees and bringing your feet back to the mat. Place your feet in front of you, keeping your knees bent, and slowly roll down onto your back to get ready for the Corkscrew.

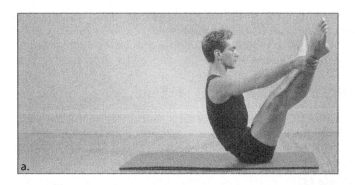

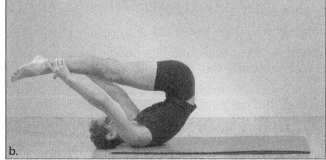

Figure 7-10:
Open Leg
Rocker.

Corkscrew

Corkscrew is an advanced variation of Rollover (an exercise from earlier in this chapter); it's basically a Rollover with a twist. So if you're pretty comfortable doing the Rollover, then go ahead and try this fun variation. Like the Rollover, the Corkscrew targets the powerhouse (your abs, inner thighs, and butt) while stretching your back and improving balance and control. The twisting aspect of this exercise demands an extra element of control.

This exercise may be difficult if you have tight hamstrings or a tight back. Also, lifting your hips up over your head is always difficult if you have a large lower body (butt). If this exercise is hard for you, practice the C Curve Roll Down Prep (Chapter 4) and the Rollover (this chapter) until you gain more strength.

Getting set

Lie down on the mat with your legs straight up to the sky in the Pilates First Position and your arms down by your sides, pressing onto the mat (Figure 7-11a).

The exercise

Inhale: Breathe in deeply, expanding your back and lungs.

Exhale: Pull your navel in toward your spine as you circle your legs to the left, down around, and back to complete the circle at the top, accenting the movement back up to the center. Keep the circles as small as necessary to maintain stability. Figures 7-11b, 7-11c, and 7-11d show the circle being made.

Inhale: Reverse the direction of the circle.

Complete 6 repetitions, alternating directions after each circle. Finish by bringing your knees into your chest and gently circling your knees, releasing the lower back.

Do's and don'ts

- ✔ Do keep your Abdominal Scoop throughout the exercise.
- ✔ Do use your arms to help you stabilize by pushing them into the mat.
- ✔ Do minimize the tension in your upper body; keep your neck long and relaxed and your back wide on the mat.
- ✔ Do squeeze your inner thighs together and also squeeze your butt to help stabilize the core.
- ✔ Don't allow your back to arch off the mat at all. Keep your lower back flat on the mat. Try for absolute stability.

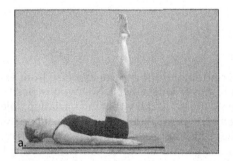
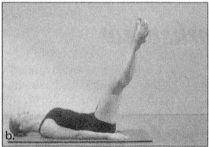
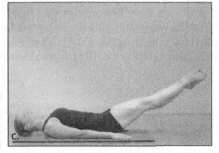
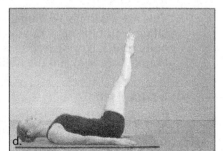

Figure 7-11:
Corkscrew.

Rising Swan

Extend your spine backward to reverse the slumping effects of sitting at a computer, watching TV, and just generally living a life on earth. Chapter 5 has the full description of Rising Swan, and Figure 7-12 shows you how to do it.

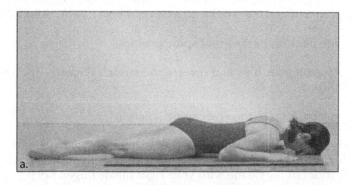

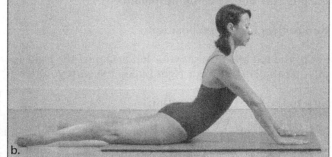

Figure 7-12: Rising Swan.

The Saw

The Saw is a great twisting stretch for your lower back. It incorporates breathing to clean out the lungs and get out all the old air. The Saw is difficult if you have tight hamstrings.

This exercise can be stressful for your lower back. Be careful if you have any serious problems with your back.

Getting set

Sit up tall with your legs straight and a little wider than the width of your hips. You can bend your legs if it's impossible for you to sit up tall with your legs straight — in other words, if you have tight hamstrings. Or you can sit on a pillow to give yourself a little lift. Reach your arms out in a T, extending your arms away from each other, palms facing down.

The exercise

Inhale: Sit up as tall as you can from the base of your spine, flex your feet, and reach through your heels to engage your leg muscles. Think of grounding your hips into the mat (Figure 7-13a).

Exhale: Lift up and out of your hips as you scoop out the low belly and twist from your waist to reach your left arm to your right calf (Figure 7-13b). Hold on to your calf and feel the stretch in your right lower back. Hold for 1 breath.

Inhale: Come back up to the erect spine position.

Exhale: Lift up off your hips and reverse the stretch (Figure 7-13c). Hold again for 1 breath.

Inhale: Come back up to the erect spine position.

Exhale: This time, instead of holding your calf, reach your right arm toward your left leg, stretching past your left foot with your hand, and think of sawing off your left pinkie toe with your right pinkie finger. Keep your right hip grounded onto the mat as a counterbalance.

Inhale: Return to the erect spine position.

Exhale: Twist to the left and stretch your left arm past the right foot, as you imagine that you're sawing off your right pinkie toe with your left pinkie finger.

Inhale: Return to the erect spine position.

Complete 3 repetitions, alternating sides, for 6 total sawing motions. Roll onto your belly for the Single Leg Kick.

Do's and don'ts

- ✔ Do keep your shoulders relaxed and down in the back.
- ✔ Don't let your hips lift off the mat when twisting. Think of reaching your opposite heel forward and grounding the opposite hip bone when stretching.
- ✔ Don't let your knees roll in as you stretch forward.

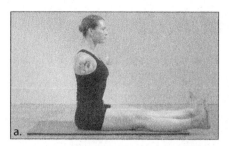

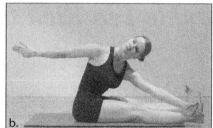

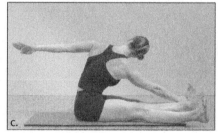

Figure 7-13:
The Saw.

Single Leg Kick

This exercise and the following one are great for your back and legs. The Single Leg Kick, from Chapter 6, is shown in Figure 7-14. Complete 10 repetitions, alternating legs each time. Finish by coming back down onto your belly, bringing your head to one side, and allowing your hands to interlace behind your back. Now you're ready to flow into the Double Leg Kick.

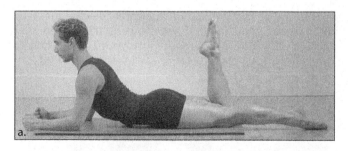

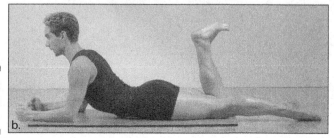

Figure 7-14:
Single Leg
Kick.

Double Leg Kick and Rest

The Double Leg Kick, from Chapter 6, is shown in Figure 7-15. Complete 4 repetitions and press back to the rest position.

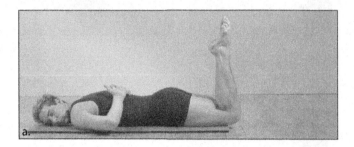

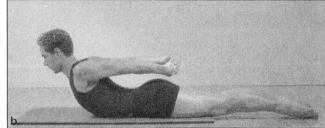

Figure 7-15:
Double Leg
Kick.

The rest position (Figure 7-16) isn't really an exercise, but a position that enables you to relax and release the back.

Sit on your heels and stretch your body forward onto the mat with your arms extended out in front of you. Imagine your lower back lengthening and releasing as your belly hollows inward. Breathe into your back. When you feel ready, roll down onto your back to get ready for the Neck Pull.

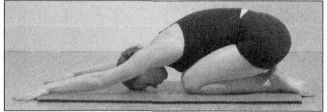

Figure 7-16:
The rest
position.

Neck Pull

The Neck Pull is one of the most difficult abdominal exercises in the mat series. When I teach this exercise to my teachers-in-training (who are quite strong!), most of them try it and shake their head, moaning, "This is impossible." And I smile, nod knowingly, and respond, "Just keep trying, and one day it will all come together." And of course, eventually it does.

The Neck Pull is a more advanced version of the Roll Up. The main difference is that in the Neck Pull, your arms remain behind your neck instead of reaching forward as they do in the Roll Up. This variation increases the load on your abdominals. Also, in the Neck Pull your legs are hip distance apart instead of being pulled together in the Pilates First Position like the Roll Up. This position also makes it harder for your abdominals because you can't help out with your butt muscles when your legs are apart. Make sure that you can do the Roll Up with control and mastery before attempting the Neck Pull. Like the Roll Up, the Neck Pull increases abdominal strength and articulation of your spine.

Getting set

Lie down on your back with your hands behind your head, fingers intertwined. Your legs should be straight out ahead of you on the floor and hip distance apart (Figure 7-17a).

The exercise

Inhale: Flex your feet and ground your heels into the mat.

Exhale: Squeeze your butt, scoop your abdominals, and begin to roll up, trying to flatten your lower back onto the mat as you rise. Imagine squeezing a tangerine under your chin to lift your head, and sequentially peel your spine off the mat. Complete the movement by rounding your back forward as you pull your navel in, hollowing your belly in opposition to the forward bend, and keeping your elbows wide. Imagine that you're reaching up and over a barrel (Figures 7-17b, 7-17c, and 7-17d show this motion).

Inhale: Stack up your spine, one vertebra at a time (your head should be the last thing to rise). Sit up tall, lifting the crown of your head to the sky, and keep your elbows wide (Figure 7-17e).

Exhale: Initiate the roll down by squeezing your butt, scooping your belly, and reaching long through your heels. Begin to roll down your spine, pulling your navel in, creating a C Curve with your lower back, and controlling the movement from the center. Think of pressing your spine down onto the mat one vertebra at a time. Roll slowly all the way down to lying flat (Figures 7-17f, 7-17g, and 7-17h show the downward movement).

Complete 5 repetitions. Finish the last one by lying flat on your back with your arms by your sides. Bend your knees and place your feet on the floor to get ready for Shoulder Bridge.

Do's and don'ts

- ✔ Do focus on using your abdominals to perform the exercise.

- ✔ Do attempt to articulate through your spine on the way down and on the way up.

- ✔ Do minimize the tension in your upper body; keep your neck long and relaxed.

- ✔ Don't yank on your neck. Allow your abdominal muscles to lift up your head.

Modification

If this exercise is too hard for you to do and you can't get up, try keeping your knees bent and your feet flat on the floor throughout the exercise, or have a friend hold down your legs.

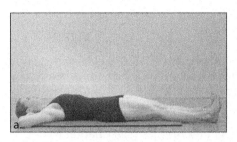

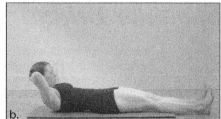

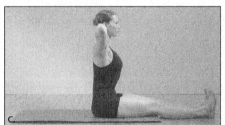

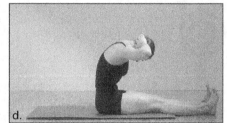

Bend forward...

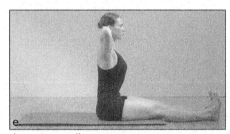

then sit up tall...

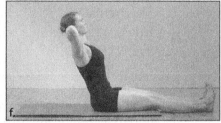

before rolling down.

Figure 7-17:
Neck Pull.

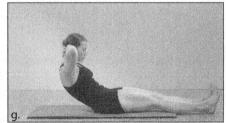

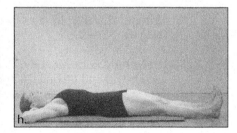

Shoulder Bridge

Shoulder Bridge is an advanced variation of Bridge. It's called Shoulder Bridge because in order to lift one leg high up off the mat while in a Bridge position, you need to be balanced up on your shoulders. This means that your hips are really lifted! Like Bridge, Shoulder Bridge strengthens your butt and the back of your legs and teaches core stability. You can warm up for this advanced version by doing a set of 3 beginner Bridges (see Chapter 5).

If you need to, prop yourself up with your arms under your hips once you get in the Bridge position.

Getting set

Lie on your back with your knees bent and your feet flat on the floor, approximately hip distance apart. Your feet should be in a comfortable position — not too close to your butt and not too far away (Figure 7-18a). Place your arms at your sides.

The exercise

Exhale: Press into your feet and squeeze your butt as you lift your back up off the mat (Figure 7-18b).

Inhale: Hold this Bridge position.

Exhale: Lift one leg off the mat, stretching it straight up while pointing your foot toward the sky (Figure 7-18c). Think of knitting your ribs down to your belly as you squeeze your butt and try to lengthen through the front of your hips.

Inhale: Lower your leg down to the height of your hips and flex your foot (Figure 7-18d).

Breathing continuously: Reach your leg back up again, pointing the foot as you go up and flexing the foot as you come down, 3 more times before you place your foot down on the mat and switch sides.

Complete 6 repetitions, alternating legs. Finish with both feet on the floor, rolling slowly down your spine, one vertebra at a time. Use the Abdominal Scoop to press your lower back onto the mat as you come back to Neutral Spine. Transition by bringing your knees into your chest to relax your back. Put one hand on each knee and slowly roll up to a sitting position. Straighten your legs out in front of you to get ready for the Spine Twist.

Do's and don'ts

✔ Do keep your belly scooped in and your butt squeezing throughout the exercise.

✔ Do reach long out of your hips as you lift and lower your leg.

✔ Don't let your hips sink. Instead, use your butt and hamstrings to press your hips up high.

✔ Don't lift your hips up so high that you put too much strain on your neck or your lower back.

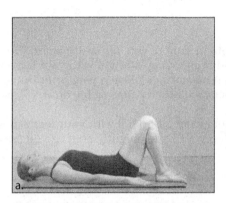
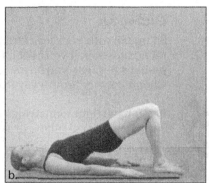
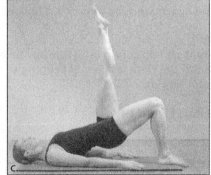
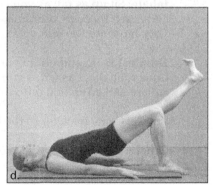

Figure 7-18: Shoulder Bridge.

Spine Twist

Twisting is a lovely way to bring flexibility back to your spine. When you twist your spine, the discs in between the vertebrae *(intervertebral discs)* become compressed. When you untwist, there is a release of compression, which is thought to allow increased fluid to flow into these spaces. Because you can easily injure yourself when twisting during daily life activities, doing these twisting exercises in a controlled setting will increase the range of motion in your spine and keep you from hurting yourself when you twist around to grab a map from the back seat of your car!

Getting set

Sit up tall with your legs straight in front of you, hip width apart. (You can bend them, however, if you absolutely can't sit up straight with your legs straight, perhaps because you have tight hamstrings.) Reach your arms out in a T, extending your arms away from each other, palms facing down (Figure 7-19a).

If you have tight hamstrings and can't sit up tall with your legs straight, try sitting on a small pillow or keep your knees slightly bent as you perform this exercise.

The exercise

Inhale: Sit up as tall as you can from the base of your spine and flex your feet and reach through your heels to engage your leg muscles. Think of grounding your hips into the mat.

Exhale: Lift up and out of your hips as you scoop out your low belly and twist from your waist as far as you can to the right while still keeping your hips square and grounded onto the mat (Figure 7-19b).

Inhale: Come back up to the center (Figure 7-19c).

Exhale: Lift up off your hips and reverse the direction of the twist (Figure 7-19d).

Inhale: Come back up to the erect spine position.

Complete 3 repetitions.

Do's and don'ts

- ✔ Do keep your shoulders relaxed and down in the back.
- ✔ Don't let your hips lift off the mat when twisting. Think of reaching your opposite heel forward and grounding the opposite hip bone when stretching.
- ✔ Don't let your knees roll in as you stretch forward.

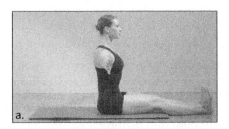
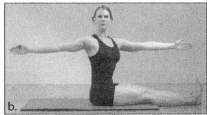
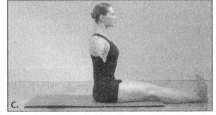
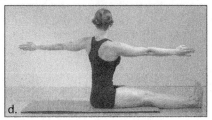

Figure 7-19:
Spine Twist.

Return to the center...   before twisting in the other dirrction.

The Jackknife

The Jackknife is similar to the Rollover, but this exercise has a percussive blast of levitation that makes it more challenging to control. Levitation, one of the letters of the Pilates alphabet (Chapter 3), is the magical lifting of the hips by the work of the powerhouse (your abdominals, butt, and inner thighs).

Skip this exercise entirely if you're not confident that you can pull it off safely, without putting too much pressure on your neck. If you do feel any strain on your neck, please don't continue.

Warm up your neck and back properly before attempting this exercise; that means do the previous exercises in the advanced series first. Please don't plop down cold and attempt this exercise! Like the Rollover, the Jackknife demands a great amount of core strength, while giving you a great stretch for your back and neck muscles. If you have problems getting your hips up and over your head (if you have a heavy bottom or tight lower back), then you may have problems with this exercise. Go back to the fundamental part of this exercise, the Hip-Up (Chapter 4), and practice that instead.

Getting set

Lie flat on your back, with your arms down by your sides, your palms facing down, and your legs straight up in the air in the Pilates First Position (Figure 7-20a). Your legs should be slightly turned out from the top of your hips, your knees should face away from each other, and your inner thighs and heels are squeezing together.

The exercise

Inhale: Take a deep breath in.

Exhale: Squeeze your butt, pull your belly in, and lift your legs up and over your head. Your legs should stop once they're parallel to the floor. Don't roll onto your neck, but stop and balance on your shoulders instead.

Inhale: Press your arms onto the floor and levitate your hips upward, reaching your toes to the sky (Figure 7-20b). Squeeze your butt and pull the belly in to accomplish this. This movement should have an explosive force to it, but with control. Be careful not to roll too high onto your neck, keeping the weight on your shoulders instead.

Exhale: Begin rolling down your spine, pressing your palms and arms on the floor to control the movement (Figure 7-20c). Try to maintain Levitation as much as possible as you roll down your spine; use your butt and belly to control the movement. Maintaining Levitation as you roll down the spine is the hard part of this exercise; it means that you try to keep your hips and legs lifting as much as possible as you roll down instead of folding in your hips.

Inhale: Lower your legs toward the mat, using your Abdominal Scoop and squeezing your butt to help you keep your lower back flat on the mat. Don't let your lower back arch off the mat even a little as you lower your legs! Lower your legs, but only low enough to still maintain your scoop and your flattened lower back. Squeeze your inner thighs together and begin the sequence again.

Complete 3 repetitions.

End by bending your knees into your chest. Roll onto your side for the next exercise, Side Kicks.

Do's and don'ts

- ✔ Do keep the movement flowing and controlled.

- ✔ Do keep your inner thighs squeezing together in the Pilates First Position and keep squeezing your butt and pulling your belly in to control the movements throughout the exercise.

- ✔ Don't let your shoulders hunch up by your ears. Instead, keep pulling your shoulder blades down your back and reaching your fingers long away from you.

- ✔ Don't roll up onto your neck. Think of keeping your neck long and the weight of your body on your shoulders.

Modifications

If you're up for a real challenge, you can do what I call the J variation of the Jackknife. Start the exercise the same way as the regular Jackknife, but instead of bringing your legs all the way overhead and parallel to the floor behind you, levitate immediately after your legs pass the 90-degree angle to the floor and make a J shape with your whole body. In other words, you don't do the explosive Jackknife movement, but instead, you flow into the J shape through smooth levitation and try to maintain this shape as you roll back down your spine. Wowee . . . feel the burn!

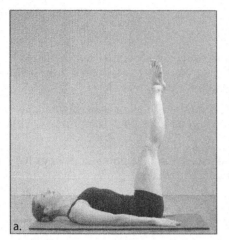
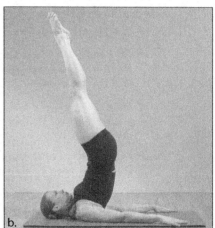
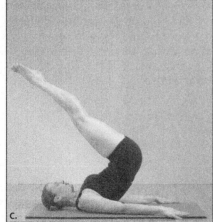

Figure 7-20:
The
Jackknife.

Side Kicks

I describe how to do Side Kicks in Chapter 5. They're a crucial exercise in the Pilates repertoire. See Figure 7-21 if you need a visual reminder of how to do them. Complete 10 repetitions, and if you want more butt and thigh work, see variations of Side Kicks in Chapter 9. Roll over onto your back to transition to the Teaser.

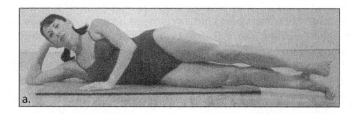

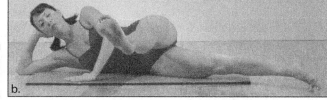

Figure 7-21:
Side Kicks.

Teaser, Advanced Version

I hope that you've already mastered the intermediate version of the Teaser before trying this one (see Chapter 6 for a description). The two versions are basically the same except that in the advanced version (which, by the way, is the "real" Teaser) the legs remain straight throughout the exercise. Also, instead of starting by sitting up in the Balance Point position as you do in the intermediate version, you start by lying on the mat. Like the intermediate Teaser, the advanced Teaser strengthens the deep abdominal muscles and increases balance and control. I think that this is one of the hardest abdominal exercises in the Pilates method!

If you find this version too hard, bend your legs and keep practicing the intermediate version in Chapter 6. Someday it will all come together!

Getting set

Lie on your back with both legs straight up to the sky in the Pilates First Position, slightly turned out from the top of the hips, your inner thighs and heels squeezing together, and your knees facing away from each other.

The exercise

Inhale: Reach your arms straight back, up by your ears, palms facing upward, and allow your legs to drop down a few inches toward the floor (Figure 7-22a).

Exhale: Keeping your arms on the floor, open them to the side, going through a T shape as you sweep your arms down by your sides. Feel your shoulder blades pulling down your back as you reach your arms forward and begin to roll up your spine. Allow your legs to drop a few more inches as you roll up. Use your Abdominal Scoop and squeeze your butt to help raise yourself up, reaching forward and up with your arms and rolling all the way up to the Teaser position, your arms parallel to your legs. Don't roll so high up that you pass your Balance Point, but instead stay balanced slightly behind your tailbone, feeling a hollow low belly and keeping a slightly rounded lower back. If you roll too far, your lower back will straighten, and you will no longer be able to feel your Abdominal Scoop. Holding the correct Balance Point position with the legs straight is what makes this exercise advanced (Figure 7-22b).

Inhale: Hold the Teaser position.

Exhale: Keep your arms reaching forward and up as you begin to roll down your spine, keeping your legs straight in the Pilates First Position. Pull your navel in and control the movement from the center. Roll slowly down until you're lying flat on the mat. Allow your arms to trail you, and as you lie down, let your arms open to a T shape on the floor as they circle back around to finish long overhead to begin again.

Complete 5 repetitions. Finish by rolling onto your belly for a Hip Flexor Stretch.

Do's and don'ts

- ✔ Do focus on using your abdominals to perform the exercise.
- ✔ Do attempt to articulate through your spine on the way down and on the way up.
- ✔ Do minimize the tension in your upper body; keep your neck long and relaxed.
- ✔ Don't continue if you can't control your movements. Instead, go back to the Balance Point exercise.

Modifications

These modifications are extremely difficult and put a lot of load on the lower back. Please stop if you feel strain there.

More difficult: Start in the same way, but instead of rolling up with the arms sweeping down by your sides, reach your arms straight up to the sky and try to keep your arms by your ears as you roll up. On the way down, use the same theory, and keep your arms by your ears as you roll down (Figure 7-22c). The extra weight of your arms in this position increases the abdominal strength necessary to complete the movement.

Even more difficult: Once you're up in the Teaser position, keep your breathing continuous as you lower your legs 6 inches and pulse them back up, using your belly to lift them up 3 times in a row.

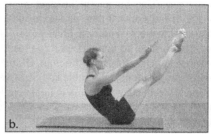

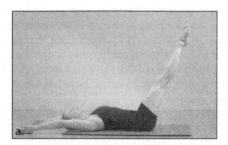

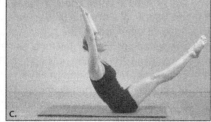

Figure 7-22:
Teaser,
Advanced
Version.

Why the psoas are pso important

Pilates instructors and dancers are obsessed with the psoas muscles. You can imagine as a dancer you do a lot of lifting up of the leg. As a Pilates instructor, you do a lot of sit-ups. Both of these motions use the psoas. Some woman actually wrote a whole book just on the psoas and ascribed emotional and psychic power to them. You may ask, "Why?"

Well, the *psoas* are the major hip flexors, connecting the legs to the torso, which means they are responsible for bringing your legs up toward your torso when you're standing or lying and for bringing your torso up to sitting when you're lying down. Dancers do a lot of lifting up of the leg, and Pilates practitioners do a lot of sit-ups. Both of these movements depend on the psoas.

The psoas are not easy to find on your body; they run so deep that you have to push through all your internal organs to feel them. I've had my psoas released before by my masseuse, and believe me, you don't want to find them — they hurt!

When you do a full sit-up from lying down on the mat, you're using not only your abdominals but also your psoas. The abdominals function to flex the torso, or round the back forward. In order to come fully up from lying down, the abdominals work in the first part of the movement (lifting the head off the mat and rounding the spine forward). The psoas works to finish the sit-up. In an exercise like the Teaser, where the legs are suspended in the air, the psoas work overtime

(continued)

(continued)

to maintain the legs up in the air and also to lift the torso up into that position. The abdominals are also working, but only in the initial rolling-up phase of the exercise; the psoas do the lion's share of the work. When you do any exercise in which you have to support your legs without moving your torso from the mat (Hundred, Single Leg Stretch, and Double Leg Stretch, for example), you use your psoas to hold your legs up while your abdominals work to keep your torso stable.

The psoas attach to the lower back, so if you feel excessive strain in your lower back while doing abdominal exercises, chances are that your psoas are being overloaded and pulling on your lower back. This can cause injury! As your abdominals get stronger and your psoas get stronger, your lower back shouldn't feel strained. But until then, don't push yourself or your psoas too hard. You never want to feel any excessive strain in your lower back when doing abdominal exercises. If you do, rest and try the modification or go back to the easier version of the exercise.

On an emotional level, some have attributed tight or sore psoas to excessive fear that's not being expressed. One writer I know theorizes that humans' only instinctual fear is the fear of falling (apes feared falling out of trees). And if you fell out of a tree, guess which muscles would work to stop the fall? Yep, you guessed it: the psoas. Because they are the central flexor of the body, the psoas stop us from falling flat on our faces. The theory goes that people who have internalized fear may unconsciously tighten their psoas, like some primordial holding pattern that, in turn, causes lower back pain.

On a more mundane level, the psoas can get tight in the average Joe Shmoe office worker. Why? Well, think about what you do at a desk. You sit. And you sit. And you sit. And what position are you in when you sit? You're in *hip flexion;* your thighs are at a 90-degree angle to the torso. In other words, the psoas are sitting in a shortened position all day long. Once 5:00 rolls around and Joe Shmoe gets up to go home, his psoas are probably tight. Believe me, in an age of sedentary work habits, most people have a tight psoas, which can eventually cause lower back problems.

If, when you try some psoas-intensive Pilates exercises like the Teaser, you feel your lower back strain, stop and lie down on your back, bring your knees up to your chest, and release the back. See the Hip Flexor Stretch exercise in this chapter for one way to stretch your poor little psoas.

Hip Flexor Stretch

Lie on your belly and bend your left leg, grabbing your left foot with your left hand. Reach your right arm out in front of you on the mat (Figure 7-23a). To increase the intensity of the stretch, try lifting your left thigh as high off the mat as possible by pulling your left foot up with your hand and pressing away with your left foot. Also, pull your navel in toward your spine and squeeze your butt, trying as hard as you can to tuck your pelvis under. You should feel a deep stretch in the front of your hip. Breathe deeply for 4 or 5 breaths, trying to increase the stretch on every exhale. Switch sides and repeat the stretch (Figure 7-23b). Roll over onto your back, propping yourself up on your elbows for Hip Circles.

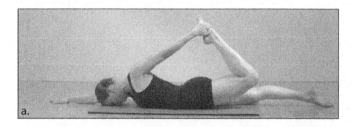

Figure 7-23: Hip Flexor Stretch.

Hip Circles

Hip Circles focus on strengthening the core muscles while stretching the chest and shoulders. Like the Teaser, Hip Circles put a load on the psoas muscles, which may strain your lower back if you're not strong enough. If your back hurts, stop and lie down on your back with your knees on your chest to release the back.

Getting set

A picture is worth a thousand words! This is a hard position to describe, so I urge you to look at Figure 7-24a. You're basically in the Balance Point position, slightly behind the tailbone, your legs straight and reaching up at a diagonal to the floor. You're propped up on your elbows and resting on your forearms behind you, with your palms facing down. Allow your legs to turn out slightly in the Pilates First Position, with your knees facing away from each other and your inner thighs and heels squeezing together.

The exercise

Inhale: Circle your legs down and around to the left, scooping your lower belly in (Figure 7-24b).

Exhale: Complete the circle, bringing your legs around to the right and back up to the starting position (Figures 7-24c and 7-24d). Accent the movement on the way back up. Keep your torso stable.

Switch directions, inhaling on the way down and exhaling on the way up.

Complete 6 repetitions.

Do's and don'ts

- ✔ Do focus on using your abdominals to perform the exercise.
- ✔ Do keep your chest lifted and your head lengthened up and out of your neck.
- ✔ Don't let your shoulders hunch up by your ears. Instead, keep your shoulder blades pulling down your back.
- ✔ Don't allow your torso to move.

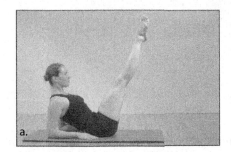
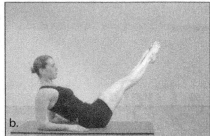
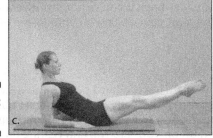
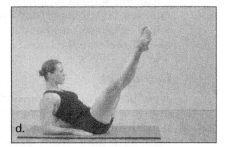

Figure 7-24:
Hip Circles.

Swimming

Whenever you start an exercise by lying on your stomach, you can be pretty sure that you'll be working the muscles of the back. So it's okay to feel the back working, but not straining.

Getting set

Lie flat on your belly with your arms stretched out in front of you and legs outstretched behind you (Figure 7-25a). Squeeze your inner thighs and heels together, in the Pilates First Position. If this position feels too compressive on your lower back, allow your legs to open slightly but still keep them turned out, with your heels dropped toward each other and your knees facing away from each other.

The exercise

Breathing continuously: Pull your navel up off the mat and raise your upper back and head off the mat slightly as you simultaneously lift your right arm and your left leg off the mat (Figure 7-25b). Squeeze your butt and try to keep pressing your pubic bone down to the mat.

Switch arms and legs and begin an even rhythm of swimming, alternating arms and legs (Figure 7-25c). Think of reaching your arms and legs long away from yourself, extending your body as much as possible.

Swim continuously for a total of 24 beats.

Finish by pressing back to the rest position, sitting on your heels to release your back (Figure 7-26). Come up to your plank position (as if you were about to do a push-up) to get ready for Control Front.

Do's and don'ts

- ✔ Do keep stretching your limbs long in opposite directions.
- ✔ Do keep squeezing your butt and pulling your navel up off the mat to protect your lower back.
- ✔ Don't let your shoulders hunch up by your ears. Instead, keep your shoulder blades pulling down your back. You may need to widen your arm width to accomplish this.
- ✔ Don't crane your head upward, but think of lengthening the back of your neck.

Modification

To make Swimming easier, don't lift your upper body and head up very high and keep your arms and legs very low and close to the mat. The higher you lift up your limbs and upper body, the more work for your butt and back muscles.

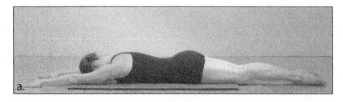

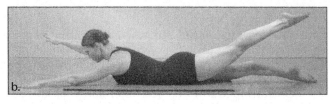

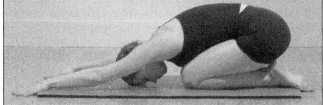

Figure 7-25:
Swimming.

Figure 7-26:
Rest
Position.

Control Front

Control Front requires a fair amount of upper body strength. The exercise focuses on strengthening the shoulders, back, and butt and increasing control and balance.

Getting set

Get into a push-up position: Place your hands shoulder distance apart and support your body on strong, straight arms. Squeeze your inner thighs together while lifting your belly and squeezing your butt. Make sure that your body is in a straight line, rigid and strong like a plank. If you feel strain in your lower back, think of lifting up your hips slightly, scooping your belly in, and really squeezing your butt. Figure 7-27a shows the correct position.

Feeling pain in your wrist?

The fundamental Pilates exercises focus on your belly, butt, and core stability. As you progress in the Pilates method, the exercises start to focus more on upper body strength. The theory goes that once you can attain core stability, supporting the weight of your body is much easier. When first attempting some of the upper body exercises that put weight on your hands, you may feel a load on your wrist. As you get stronger in your back and shoulders, you won't feel the stress on your wrist as much.

Here are some tips to get the load off the wrist:

✔ Keep your wrist aligned with your shoulder. In other words, your fingers should point in the same direction as your upper arm. If you're in a plain push-up position or plank, your fingers should point forward. If your arm is turned out to one side, your fingers should also point out in that direction.

✔ Practice cupping the palm to lift the weight off the actual wrist crease. Spread your fingers and think of pressing away the floor with all your finger muscles, especially your thumb and pinkie, and try to lift the weight off your central palm and wrist area.

✔ Keep thinking of lifting the weight out of your wrist by pressing away from the floor by using your back and shoulder muscles.

✔ Try a hard surface. Performing exercises that put weight on your hands is easier on the wrist when done on a hard surface, such as a wooden floor, rather than on a mat or a rug. The harder surface allows for more stability in your hand and wrist joint and makes it easier to press away from gravity.

You're a wooden plank that could withstand weight if someone were to step up on your back.

The exercise

Breathing continuously: Maintain your plank position and rock forward and back on your toes 4 times (Figure 7-27b). Keep your torso stable by pulling in your belly by using your Abdominal Scoop and squeezing your butt.

Keeping the rhythm of the rocking, lift your right leg up and hold it there as you rock forward and back 3 times (Figure 7-27c). Point and flex the foot of your lifted right leg, as shown in Figure 7-27d, as you mirror the rocking on the left foot (as you rock forward, point the foot; as you rock backward, flex the foot). Put your foot back down as you rock forward, and switch legs.

Complete 6 repetitions, alternating legs. Finish by bending your knees and coming to a kneeling position for Kneeling Side Kicks.

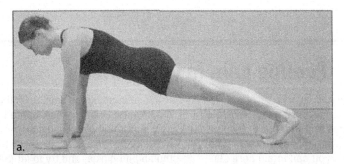

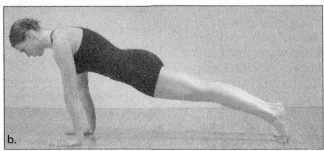

Rock forward and back.

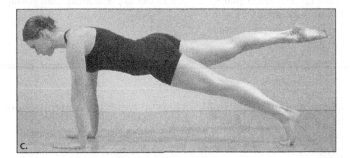

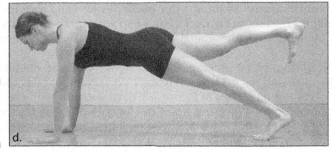

Figure 7-27:
Control
Front.

Do's and don'ts

- Do keep the crown of your head reaching long in front of you.

- Do keep squeezing your butt and pulling your navel in by using your Abdominal Scoop throughout the exercise.

- Don't let your shoulders hunch up by your ears. Instead, keep your shoulder blades pulling down your back.

Modification

You'll gain upper body and core strength just by holding the plank position. After you can hold the plank for 10 seconds, try adding the rocking forward and back on your toes.

Kneeling Side Kicks

This exercise is an advanced version of Side Kicks, which you can find pictured back in Figure 7-21 and described in detail in Chapter 5. Being up on your knees rather than lying on your side increases the balance and control necessary to accomplish the exercise.

Getting set

Kneeling on the front edge of your mat, place one hand on the mat directly below your shoulder, turning the hand outward, so the fingers are pointing in the same direction as your head (your fingers parallel to the side edge of the mat). Place your other hand behind your head. Lift your top leg to the height of your hips and straighten it long away from you. Keep your hips pressing forward so that your whole body — knees, hips, shoulders, and outstretched leg — is on one plane (Figure 7-28).

The exercise

Inhale: Kick your top leg straight out in front of you, flexing your foot and trying not to break at your waist. Keep pushing your hips forward by squeezing your butt and pulling your navel in toward your spine.

Exhale: Kick your leg behind you, pointing your foot and keeping it the same height as your hip. Try not to let your back arch. Squeeze your butt and pull your navel in to help stabilize.

Compete 10 repetitions, come back up to kneeling, and turn to the other side.

Transition by sitting on your heels and go on to the Sidebend/Advanced Mermaid.

Do's and don'ts

 ✔ Do press your weight into the front palm on the floor to maintain balance throughout the exercise.

 ✔ Do keep your neck long and relaxed.

 ✔ Do keep your body square, shoulder over shoulder and hip over hip.

 ✔ Don't wobble like a noodle. Maintain stability in your body as your leg moves freely, especially when kicking to the back. Keep your hips square to the front throughout the exercise.

Modification

To simplify the exercise, keep the leg movement as small as necessary in the beginning and make stability of your body the main concern. Increase the movement of your leg to the back and front as you gain the core strength.

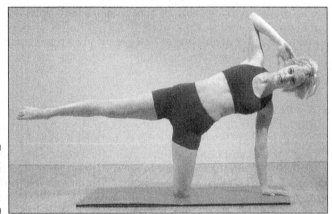

Figure 7-28:
Kneeling
Side Kicks.

Side Bend/Advanced Mermaid

This exercise really works your back and shoulder muscles *(latissimus dorsi)*, while giving you a lovely stretch all along the side of your body.

Getting set

Start in the mermaid position: Sit on the side of your hip, propped up on a straight arm, your fingers facing away from you, your knees bent, your ankles close together, and your top foot in front (Figure 7-29a).

The exercise

Inhale: Press into the arm that's on the floor and come up into a side plank lifting your hips up and stretching your arm overhead close to your top ear

(Figure 7-29b). Keep your supporting shoulder strong and stable in the back while holding your weight up with that arm, thinking of pressing away from the floor from your back muscles.

VISUALIZE

Your body is like a wooden plank, strong and stable.

Exhale: As your arm comes down to the starting position, drop your hips back down, almost to the floor without actually touching the floor (Figure 7-29c). You should feel a great stretch in the side of your lower back.

Inhale: Come back up to the side plank again, repeating the motion that started the exercise. Lift your hips up and stretch your arm overhead close to your top ear (Figure 7-29d). Doing this takes a great amount of shoulder strength.

Repeat the hip drop and lift 3 times. On the last repetition, come back to sitting in the mermaid position. Switch sides. Finish by scooting to the front of your mat, sitting with your knees open, and grabbing onto your ankles to transition to The Seal.

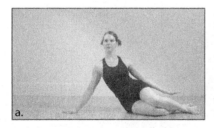
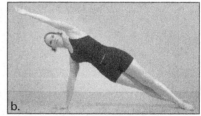
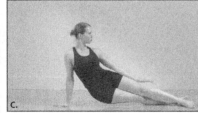
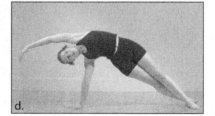

Figure 7-29:
Side Bend/
Advanced
Mermaid.

Do's and don'ts

- ✔ Do lift your hips up high to take weight off your upper body.
- ✔ Maintain stability in your shoulder when initiating the first movement.
- ✔ Do elongate your limbs as much as possible to get a great stretch.
- ✔ Don't let your shoulders hunch up by your ears.
- ✔ Don't continue if your wrist strains. Rest instead.

Modification

If you find this exercise too difficult, try coming up to the side plank and holding it for 1 breath.

The Seal

Do the Seal, which is described in Chapter 6 and shown in Figure 7-30. Complete 6 repetitions and, on the last one, try to release your hands from your feet and roll up to standing to transition to the Pilates Push-Up. This is a tough movement, but allowing your head to drop down as you roll forward, then letting your head lead you up to standing makes it easier.

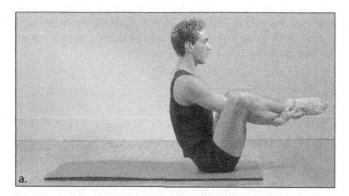

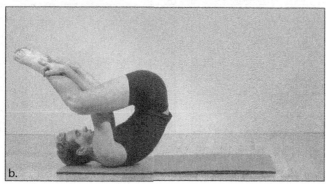

Figure 7-30:
The Seal.

Pilates Push-Up

The Pilates Push-Up combines a nice stretch and release for the back and hamstrings with a classic push-up. The exercise strengthens your shoulders, back, and butt and increases spinal articulation.

Getting set

Stand up at the back of your mat, with your legs in the Pilates First Position (slightly turned out from the top of your hips, knees facing away from each other, and inner thighs squeezing together) and your arms reaching overhead (Figure 7-31a).

The exercise

Inhale: Pull your navel in and squeeze your butt, stretching your arms high overhead like you just woke up and you're getting your first stretch of the day.

Exhale: Reach your arms forward and then down, making an arc, as you begin to roll down your spine, starting with your head dropping forward, then your neck and upper back, and finally your lower back, and come to a forward bend. Allow your arms to hang forward as you roll. Come all the way down and reach your hands to the mat in front of you (Figure 7-31b). Think of keeping your abdominals lifting up as your back goes down.

Inhale: Walk your hands out along the mat in front of you until your hands are directly beneath your shoulders (Figure 7-31c).

Exhale: Lower your hips and come into a push-up position: Place your hands shoulder distance apart and your legs together, lift your belly, and squeeze your butt. Keep your heels together. Make sure that your body is in a straight line, rigid and strong like a wooden plank (Figure 7-30d). If you feel strain in your lower back, think of lifting up your hips slightly and really squeezing your butt.

Inhaling and exhaling: Maintaining your plank position, do 8 push-ups. Inhale on the way down and exhale on the way up. Try to go slowly and with control. Keep your torso stable by pulling in your belly, using your Abdominal Scoop, and squeezing your butt (Figure 7-31e).

Inhale: Walk your hands back toward your feet and hang down in your forward bend stretch, keeping your head hanging heavy. You may need to bend your knees slightly if the stretch is too excruciating.

Exhale: Soften your knees and begin stacking up the spine, lifting your navel up and in toward your spine as if you're being lifted from the middle. Keep your head hanging heavy as you rise, stacking the spine one vertebra at a time. Finish by standing tall, your head the last thing to rise.

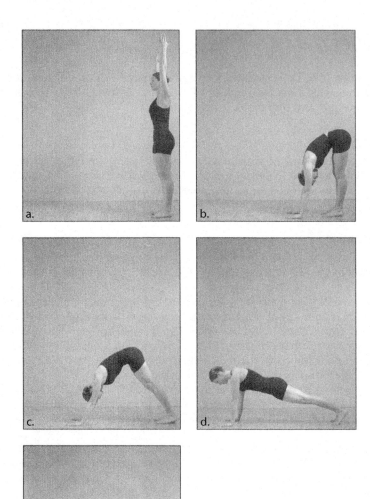

Do's and don'ts

- ✔ Do keep the crown of your head reaching long in front of you while doing the push-up.

- ✔ Do keep squeezing your butt and pulling your navel in by using your Abdominal Scoop throughout the exercise.

- ✔ Don't let your shoulders hunch up by your ears. Instead, keep your shoulder blades pulling down your back.

Modifications

You'll gain upper body and core strength just by holding the plank position. After you can hold the plank for 10 seconds, roll back up to standing.

To make the Pilates Push-Up even harder, once you get out to the plank position, lift one leg off the mat and do the push-up sequence on one leg. You may need to lift your pelvis up a little to maintain balance. Finish the sequence and repeat on the other side.

Chapter 8

Maybe Someday . . .
Super Advanced Exercises

In This Chapter

▶ Adding super advanced exercises to your program

▶ Challenging yourself to the max

*I*f you've mastered the advanced series in Chapter 7, you can challenge yourself anew with the exercises in this chapter. Some of these exercises are variations of intermediate or advanced exercises (the Super Advanced Corkscrew, for example). If this is the case, merely replace the advanced exercise with the super advanced version when you do the advanced series. Other exercises are just really, really difficult. An exercise can be considered super advanced if it takes a huge amount of strength, coordination, or control. Some super advanced exercises require all three together!

There's not really a super advanced series. Just add the exercises that aren't variations of other exercises at the end of your advanced workout, once you've properly warmed up your whole body. Good luck!

Super Advanced Exercises in This Chapter

If you're ready to take on the exercises that make even Pilates instructors wince, here they are:

- ✔ The Twist
- ✔ Control Balance
- ✔ Super Advanced Corkscrew
- ✔ Super Advanced Teaser
- ✔ Swan Dive
- ✔ The Star
- ✔ Boomerang

The Twist

The Twist requires a great deal of upper body strength and core stability. It's a great exercise for gaining strength and stability in the shoulders, and it gives your spine a lovely stretch. To prepare for this exercise, practice Side Bends/Advanced Mermaid (see Chapter 7). If you can do Side Bends with ease, then you'll have no problem with the Twist.

This exercise puts a lot of strain on the wrist. Be cautious if you have repetitive-strain or other wrist injuries.

Getting set

Sitting on the side of your hip, prop yourself up on a straight arm. Your fingers should be facing away from you with your knees bent, your ankles close together, and your top foot in front. You should be sitting like a mermaid (Figure 8-1a). Take a deep breath in.

The exercise

Exhale: Lift yourself up on the arm that's supporting you so that your body makes a side plank. Simultaneously, stretch your free arm overhead close to the top ear (Figure 8-1b). Keep your lower shoulder strong and stable, thinking of pressing away from the floor from your back muscles.

Inhale: Come to a T position, reaching your free arm up to the sky (Figure 8-1c).

Exhale: Hollow your belly and stretch your arm through the arch made by your torso. This movement, shown in Figure 8-1d, is known as threading the needle.

If the image of threading a needle doesn't work for you, think of yourself as carving out a large ball with your hand.

Inhale: Come back to a T and then increase the stretch by reaching your arm backward, opening your chest, and looking back at your arm (Figure 8-1e). All the while, maintain square hips to the front.

Exhale: Come back to the T again.

Inhale: Return to the starting position, sitting like a mermaid.

Complete 3 repetitions and switch sides for 3 more repetitions.

Do's and don'ts

  ✔ Do lift your hips up high to take your weight off your upper body.

  ✔ Do maintain stability in your shoulder when initiating the first movement.

✔ Do elongate your limbs as much as possible to get a great stretch.

✔ Don't let your shoulders hunch up by your ears.

✔ Don't continue if your wrist feels strained. Rest instead.

Modification

If you find this exercise too difficult, try just coming up to your side plank and holding it for 1 breath and then come back to the start position.

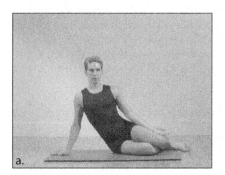

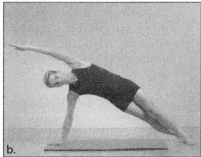

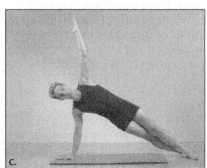

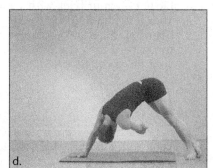

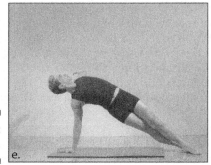

Figure 8-1:
The Twist.

Control Balance

Control Balance is my new favorite exercise to teach the essence of Levitation, which is one of the letters of the Pilates alphabet (see Chapter 3). Levitation is an advanced concept that combines a Hip-Up, a butt squeeze, and a little magic. Like the swamis in the '70s who supposedly rose up from their half lotus during deep meditation, you too can rise — with a little help from your powerhouse (your abs, inner thighs, and butt).

Control Balance requires exactly that: control and balance. You'll see when you first try this exercise that if either element is missing, you'll fall out of position. Control Balance may seem impossible at first, but keep trying, and someday it will all come together. When done correctly, Control Balance strengthens your abdominals and butt and gives you a great stretch through your whole spine.

Control Balance can put a load on your neck. Avoid this exercise if you have a neck injury.

Getting set

Lie flat on your back with your arms down by your sides, palms facing down. Your legs should be in the Pilates First Position (a letter of the Pilates alphabet from Chapter 3), straight up to the sky and slightly turned out from the top of your hips. Your knees should be facing away from each other, with your inner thighs and heels squeezing together. Take a deep breath in.

The exercise

Exhale: Press your arms onto the floor and come up to a shoulder stand, lifting your hips upward and reaching your toes to the sky (Figure 8-2a). Squeeze your butt and pull your belly in to accomplish this Levitation. Try to give the movement an explosive force while keeping it controlled. Don't roll onto your neck; stop and balance on your shoulders.

Inhale: Drop your right leg down toward your head and grab onto your calf with both hands (Figure 8-2b). While keeping a firm hold on your right calf, reach your left leg up to the sky. Use your Abdominal Scoop and squeeze your butt to keep your hips in the air and to find the inner control of the position. Pull your right calf down with a gentle *double pulse* (pull the calf down with your hands, let it rebound a bit, and pull it down again). This movement is meant to test your stability.

Make sure that you're not putting weight on your neck. If swallowing is difficult, you're up too high on your neck. In this case, roll down off your neck.

The trick to this exercise is to find the point where you can lift your top leg as high as possible while not putting stress on your neck. You must use your arm strength to hold down the lower leg in order to counter the forward pull of the lifted leg. Think of the legs splitting apart, while the lower leg is held stable.

Alternate legs, and complete 6 repetitions.

End by rolling down onto your back and bending your knees into your chest.

Do's and don'ts

- ✔ Do keep your hips lifting throughout the exercise.
- ✔ Don't let your shoulders hunch up by your ears. Keep pulling your shoulder blades down your back.
- ✔ Don't roll up onto your neck. Think of keeping your neck long and the weight of your body on your shoulders and upper back.

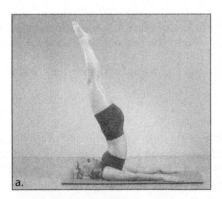
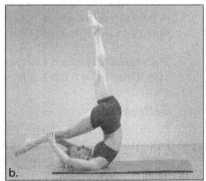
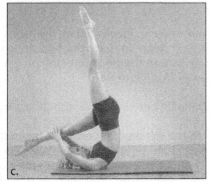

Figure 8-2:
Control
Balance.

Modification

You can keep your arms down on the floor for support while you drop your right leg down and reach your left leg up to the sky. Alternate legs and complete 6 repetitions.

Super Advanced Corkscrew

The Super Advanced Corkscrew is basically a Rollover with a twist. Like the Rollover, the Super Advanced Corkscrew targets your powerhouse while stretching your back and improving balance and control. The twisting aspect of this exercise requires you to exert an extra element of control.

This exercise may be difficult for you if you have tight hamstrings or a tight back. Also, lifting your hips up over your head is always difficult if you have a large lower body.

Before attempting this version of the Corkscrew, make sure that you have mastered the Rollover (Chapter 7) and the regular Corkscrew (Chapter 7).

The Super Advanced Corkscrew can put a load on your neck. Avoid this exercise if you have a neck injury.

Getting set

Lie down on the mat with your legs straight up to the sky in the Pilates First Position (your legs turned out from the top of your hips, and your inner thighs squeezing together). Put your arms down by your sides and press them into the mat with your palms facing down.

The exercise

Inhale: Pull your belly in, pull your inner thighs together, and squeeze your butt to lift your legs up and over your head so that your legs are parallel to the floor behind you. Push your arms into the floor to help you get your hips up. Keep your shoulders down away from your ears.

Don't roll back onto your neck; balance between your shoulder blades.

Exhale: Twist your hips slightly to the left and let your legs begin to circle down to the right. Roll down the right side of your spine. Push your arms into the floor to facilitate this movement. As you roll down your spine, allow your legs to continue the circle, dropping them down and then up to the left. Complete the circle by bringing your legs back to the center. Figure 8-3 shows the circular corkscrew-like movement.

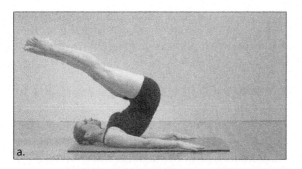

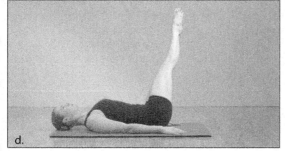

Allow your spine to roll down the mat as your legs mak
a circle.

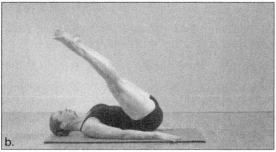

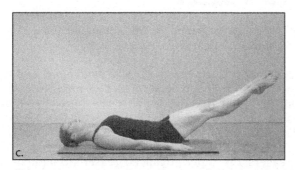

Figure 8-3:
The twisting
motion of
the Super
Advanced
Corkscrew.

When circling your legs, allow your legs to drop as close to the floor as you can without your belly pooching out or your back arching off the mat. Keep your torso stable at all costs by pulling your navel in toward your spine and squeezing your butt!

Complete 4 repetitions, alternating directions each time. Finish by bringing your knees into your chest.

Do's and don'ts

- ✔ Do keep your Abdominal Scoop throughout the exercise.
- ✔ Do use your arms to help you stabilize yourself by pushing into the mat.
- ✔ Do minimize the tension in your upper body; keep your neck long and relaxed and keep your back wide on the mat.
- ✔ Do squeeze your butt and inner thighs together to help stabilize the core.
- ✔ Don't allow your back to arch off the mat at all. Keep your lower back flat on the mat when dropping your legs toward the floor. Try for absolute stability.

Super Advanced Teaser

Okay, so you need a little more challenge. The Advanced Teaser from Chapter 7 wasn't hard enough. Well, here goes. . . .

The Super Advanced Teaser starts in what I call a *dead hang.* This means that you are outstretched on the mat and must lift all four limbs from the most difficult possible position. I think that this is one of the hardest abdominal exercises in the Pilates method. Try it, and if you can't seem to get it going, just go back to the Advanced Teaser for a while.

Like all the other Teasers, the Super Advanced Teaser strengthens the deep abdominal muscles and increases balance and control. This variation takes a huge amount of abdominal control, as well as strength in the muscles that flex the hip (the psoas).

If you feel strain in your lower back, stop and rest by lying on your back with your knees up to your chest.

Getting set

Start in your dead hang, as shown in Figure 8-4a, with your whole body extended out on the mat, your arms reaching overhead, and your legs long out in front of you in the Pilates First Position (your legs slightly turned out from the top of your hips, and your heels and inner thighs glued together). Take a deep breath in.

The exercise

Exhale: Pull your navel in and squeeze your butt as you lift your arms and legs simultaneously (Figure 8-4b) and slowly come up to your Teaser position, as shown in Figure 8-4c. Your legs are reaching diagonally up and make a V shape with your torso, your arms reach forward toward your toes, and your weight is balanced just behind your tailbone.

Inhale: Reach your arms up by your ears (Figure 8-4d) and begin to roll down your spine, allowing your legs to slowly drop toward the mat as you control the movement down. Pull your navel in and control the movement from your center. You'll end up with your arms reaching overhead and your legs long out in front of you, back to the dead hang position that you started in.

Complete 4 repetitions.

Do's and don'ts

- ✔ Do focus on using your abdominals to perform the exercise.
- ✔ Do protect your lower back by squeezing your butt and pulling your navel in toward your spine while coming up from the dead hang position.
- ✔ Do try to go slowly and control the movements on the way up and the way down.
- ✔ Do minimize the tension in your upper body; keep your neck long and relaxed.
- ✔ Don't continue if your back hurts.

Modification

To make this exercise even more difficult, once you're up in the Teaser position, lower your legs 6 inches and pulse them back up, 3 times in a row, accenting the up movement and using your belly to lift. Then roll back down to the dead hang.

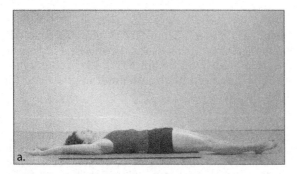

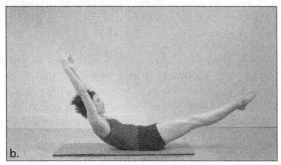

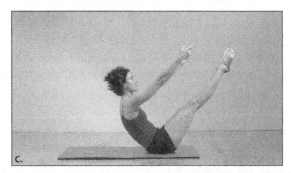

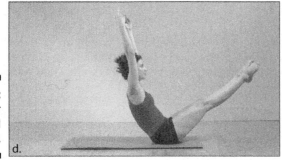

Figure 8-4:
Super
Advanced
Teaser.

Swan Dive

Swan Dive is a super advanced version of the Rising Swan from Chapter 5. You need a great amount of back flexibility to do the Swan Dive, so avoid this exercise if you suffer from an overly tight or sore lower back. Swan Dive strengthens all the muscles of the back of your body: your back and neck muscles, your butt, and your hamstrings.

Because you're rolling on the front of your body, don't do this exercise after eating or with a full bladder! Make sure that you do the Rising Swan first to warm up your back for the Swan Dive.

Getting set

Lie on your belly with your forehead flat on the mat, your arms bent, your elbows close to your side, and your palms facing down by your ears. Keeping your legs approximately hip distance apart, allow them to turn out from the top of your hips, dropping your heels toward each other.

The exercise

Inhale: Pull your navel up off the mat as if you were going to slide a piece of paper under your belly, and press your pubic bone down into the mat. Squeeze your low butt and think of lengthening out your lower back. This is your powerhouse at work!

Exhale: Straighten your arms by pressing your hands into the mat (Figure 8-5a). Protect your lower back by again pulling your belly in and squeezing your butt.

Inhale: Release your hands, reaching your chest to the sky, and roll forward onto your chest (Figure 8-5b). Stretch your arms out in front of you and lift your legs up as high as possible behind you.

Exhale: Using your momentum, rock back onto your thighs and reach your chest and arms to the sky.

Continue rocking back and forth, inhaling as you roll forward and exhaling as you roll back.

Roll back and forth a total of 4 times and sit back on your heels in the rest position. Your back will definitely need a rest after this extreme extension! The rest position allows the back to rest after all that work.

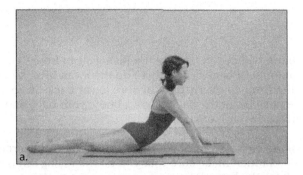

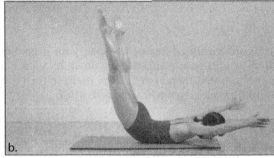

Figure 8-5:
Swan Dive.

Use your momentum as you roll
forward and backward.

Do's and don'ts

✔ Do keep your head and neck stable in this exercise. Don't let your head
rock back and forth. Think of the head and neck following the curve of
the spine.

✔ Don't continue if you feel compression or discomfort in your lower back.

The Star

You can consider this exercise a super advanced variation of Side Kicks (see
Chapter 5 for a description of Side Kicks). In the beginning version of Side
Kicks, you lie on your side and kick. In the advanced version, Kneeling Side
Kicks (Chapter 7), you kneel on your knee and kick. And in this super
advanced version, you maintain a side plank while you kick (and you add arm
movements, just for good measure).

The exercise increases in difficulty as the position from which you kick
becomes more difficult to stabilize. To master the Star, you must have a great
amount of upper body strength, as well as core and shoulder stability.

This exercise puts some strain on the wrist. Be cautious if you have repetitive-strain or other wrist injuries. Try doing this exercise on a hard surface rather than on the mat to help stabilize your wrist joint.

Getting set

Sitting on the side of your hip, prop yourself up on a straight arm, with your fingers facing away from you. Bend your knees, keep your ankles close together, and place your top foot in front. You should be sitting like a mermaid.

The exercise

Inhale: Press on your supporting arm and come to a side plank. Straighten your legs, lifting your hips up, and reach your free arm up to the sky so that your body makes the shape of a T that's fallen on its side (Figure 8-6a). Keep the lower shoulder strong and stable in the back, thinking of pressing away from the floor with your back muscles.

Exhale: Press the side edge of your bottom foot onto the floor as you raise the top leg up so that it's a little higher than your hip (Figure 8-6b).

Think of yourself as a star reaching your limbs long in all directions.

Inhale: Kick your top leg straight out in front of you, flexing your foot, and try to touch your toes by reaching forward with your top arm. Try not to break at your waist (Figure 8-6c).

Exhale: Kick your top leg behind you, pointing your foot (Figure 8-6d). Keep your leg slightly higher than your hip and try not to let your back arch. Squeeze your butt and pull your navel in for stability. As your leg moves back, your top arm reaches forward and up.

Repeat 2 more times. On the third repetition, as your leg reaches back, allow your back to arch and your chest to open. Finish by bringing your top foot down to the floor and come back to the Mermaid position.

Switch sides and complete 3 more repetitions.

Do's and don'ts

- ✔ Do lift your hips up high to take weight off your upper body.
- ✔ Do maintain stability in the shoulder of your supporting arm by thinking of pulling your shoulder blade down your back.
- ✔ Don't let your body wiggle around; keep the core stable.
- ✔ Don't continue if your wrist strains. Rest instead.

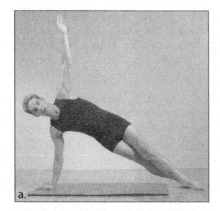
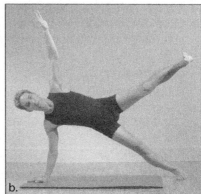
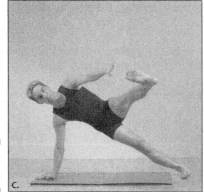
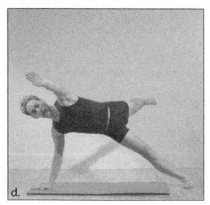

Figure 8-6:
The Star.

Modification

If you find this exercise too difficult, try just holding the star shape (Figure 8-6b) for 8 counts and come back to the mermaid position. After you gain the back strength to hold this position, you can add the movement of the leg.

Boomerang

Boomerang is one of my all-time favorite exercises because it combines many advanced Pilates concepts and skills into one flowing exercise. Within the Boomerang, you will find two Teasers (Chapters 6 and 7), a Jackknife (Chapter 7), a Rollover (Chapter 7), and a Spine Stretch Forward (Chapter 5). Boomerang requires that you have a great amount of control, balance, and coordination. When accomplished, it increases spinal articulation and core strength and stretches out the back and neck muscles.

You must be able to do a Teaser, a Jackknife, and a Rollover before attempting this exercise. If you have lower back or neck problems, avoid this exercise.

Getting set

Sit up tall with your legs straight out in front of you and your right ankle crossed over your left. Reach your arms out to the sides so that they make a T shape with your torso. Take a deep breath in.

The exercise

Try to count out the positions in your head as you do them. When you get to Step 8, you will transition seamlessly back to Step 1.

Step 1

Exhale: Roll back into the first of two Teasers that you'll do in this exercise, with your arms circling forward and reaching toward your toes, and your legs lifting up diagonally toward the sky and keeping their crossed position. You should be in your Balance Point, balancing just behind your tailbone and using your Abdominal Scoop to keep your balance (Figure 8-7a).

Step 2

Inhale: Roll back into a Jackknife by rolling back onto your spine, levitating your hips to the sky, lifting from your belly and butt, and pressing your arms down onto the mat for support. Balance between your shoulders and don't roll up onto your neck. Your legs should be straight up to the ceiling. When they reach the top, switch your legs quickly, placing your left leg in front (Figure 8-7b).

Step 3

Exhale: Allow your legs to slowly drop back behind you, stopping after they're parallel to the floor. Don't let your toes touch the floor behind you. Don't roll onto your neck; stop and balance on your shoulders. Keep pressing your arms onto the mat for support (Figure 8-7c).

Step 4

Inhale: Begin to slowly roll all the way down your spine. Think of reaching your toes long toward the wall behind you. Keep pressing your palms and arms on the floor to control the movement (Figure 8-7d).

Step 5

Exhale: Once your tailbone has touched down, allow your legs to keep moving toward the floor as you roll up into your second Teaser, reaching your arms diagonally toward your toes. Your legs, still crossed at the ankles, should make a V shape with your torso. You should be in your Balance Point, balancing just behind your tailbone and using your Abdominal Scoop to maintain the position (Figure 8-7e).

Step 6

Inhale: Holding this balance, allow your arms to swim around to the sides and then behind your back. Interlace your fingers behind your back (Figure 8-7f).

Step 7

Exhale: Keep this shape as you allow your legs to come down and rest on the mat and your back to bow forward over your legs (Figure 8-7g). Perform this movement with control — no falling with a plop!

Step 8 — back to Step 1

Inhale: Release your hands without popping them apart, and swim your arms open to the sides and forward as you roll back into your first Teaser (Figure 8-7h). You're back at Step 1!

Complete 4 repetitions.

Finish the last Boomerang by reaching your arms toward your toes with your spine rounded forward in a bow for a nice stretch.

Do's and don'ts

- ✔ Do keep the movement flowing and controlled.
- ✔ Don't plop in and out of any position; all movements must be controlled from the core.
- ✔ Don't roll up onto your neck. Think of keeping your neck long.

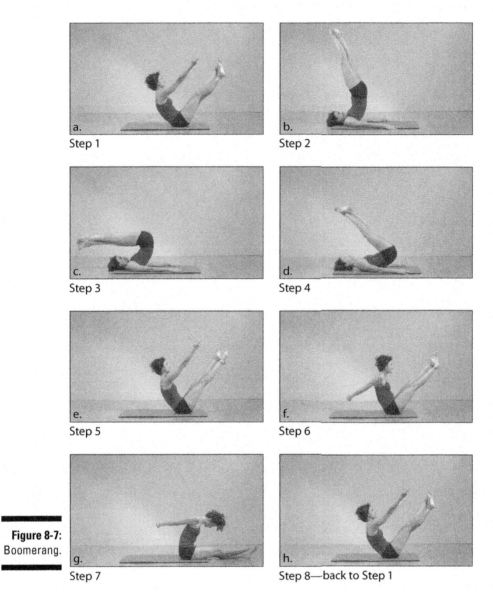

a.
Step 1

b.
Step 2

c.
Step 3

d.
Step 4

e.
Step 5

f.
Step 6

Figure 8-7:
Boomerang.

g.
Step 7

h.
Step 8—back to Step 1

Chapter 9

Extra Help for the Butt and Thighs

In This Chapter

▶ Toning and shaping your butt and thighs

▶ Working on the Side Kick series

Do you dream of slimmer hips and a firmer butt? Who doesn't? I can't promise you a completely new body, but I can assure you that if you spend ten minutes a day focusing on the exercises in this chapter, you'll see a difference in the tone and shape of your thighs and butt.

Vanity isn't the only reason to check out this chapter; having a strong butt is essential to stabilize the pelvis when running, walking, skiing, or doing anything on your legs. Strong butt muscles also protect your back from overuse, and thus can alleviate back pain.

Simply add these exercises to your series when you get to the Side Kicks exercise (the beginning, intermediate, and advanced series all have the Side Kicks exercise included in them). Doing so increases the difficulty of the series and really makes your butt and thighs work hard.

Engaging Your Butt

The butt is made up of three muscles: the gluteus maximus, the gluteus medius, and the gluteus minimus. All three help to stabilize your pelvis when you walk, and when weak, they can cause lower back pain or a number of other problems. The gluteus maximus is the main fleshy part of your butt, and the gluteus medius and minimus are both on the side of your butt, right behind your hipbones.

I want to focus on the gluteus maximus, which I normally just call the glut max. As you can tell by its name, it's the biggest butt muscle. It makes up much of what you consider to be your butt. Isolating the glut max can be hard, so knowing when it's doing its thing is important.

The glut max has two main functions: to stabilize the pelvis when you're moving around and to move the thigh backward. Anytime you bring your leg behind your body (called *hip extension*), you should be using your gluteus maximus. To ensure that you're working the glut max as much as possible when doing Pilates, don't arch your back as your leg goes behind you. This advice applies to exercises you do while lying on your belly and to exercises you do while lying on your side, like all the variations of Side Kicks that are in this chapter.

If your back arches when you extend your hip, you're using your back muscles and aren't effectively stabilizing with your butt. Your butt works only when the leg is no more than 15 degrees behind your body. If you move your leg back any more than that, you're arching your back and using your back muscles. So if you want to isolate the glut max, you must limit how far you kick your leg behind you (don't go more than 15 degrees back).

Always think of squeezing the butt and using your Abdominal Scoop to help you stabilize your back and pelvis and to stop you from arching your back when extending your leg behind you. You can apply this thought to every step you take, literally. When you walk, think of walking from your hips rather than from your knees — you'll use your butt more. Imagine that someone's hands are on your butt pushing you forward as you stride.

Butt and Thigh Exercises in This Chapter

Here's a preview of the butt and thigh exercises in this chapter. Together, they make the Side Kick series:

- ✔ Side Kicks
- ✔ Bicycle
- ✔ Up/Down in Parallel
- ✔ Butt Cruncher
- ✔ Inner Thigh Pulses
- ✔ Up/Down in Turnout
- ✔ Up/Down with Passé
- ✔ Figure 8
- ✔ Grande Ronde de Jambe

Getting Started On the Side Kick Series

The exercises in this chapter comprise the Side Kick series. Try to do all the exercises in a row; they're meant to follow each other. If you can complete the whole series, you'll definitely feel a delicious burn all around your butt.

Please note that some exercises in the Side Kick series are more advanced than others. If you come to an exercise in this series that feels too advanced for you, skip it and move on to the next one. I state the difficulty of the exercise next to its name.

You do a lot of flexing and pointing of the feet in this chapter, so I thought I'd remind you what the terms mean. You're flexing your foot when you pull your toes back up toward your legs. You're pointing your foot when you reach your toes away from you.

Go through the series on one side and then flip over and do the series lying on your other side.

Side Kicks (Beginning)

It's no surprise that the classic Side Kick series starts with Side Kicks. If you've done the series in Chapters 5, 6, or 7, you've done Side Kicks already. They're described in full in Chapter 5. Try doing the advanced variation, where both your hands are behind your head. Figure 9-1 shows Side Kicks, and Figure 9-2 shows the advanced hand position.

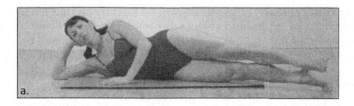

a.

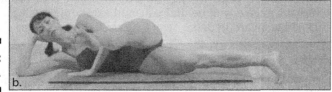

Figure 9-1:
Side Kicks.

b.

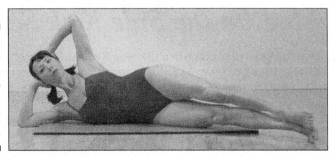

Figure 9-2:
Make Side Kicks more difficult by changing your hand position.

Bicycle (Beginning)

In this exercise, you move your legs like you're riding a bike — only you're lying on your side.

Getting set

Lie on your side, propped up on one elbow with the hand supporting your head. Place your other hand behind your head. Your legs should be together and slightly in front of your body. Keep your hips square during the exercise. Point your knees straight ahead (as opposed to facing slightly away from each other), in what is known as the parallel position. Point your feet. (Figure 9-3a shows the starting position.)

If you're struggling with this exercise, put the palm of your top arm on the mat for support.

The exercise

Breathing continuously: Lift your top leg up slightly so that it's even with your hips. Point your foot and swing your top leg forward as far as you can while still maintaining stability in your torso (Figure 9-3b), and then bend your knee as if you are pedaling a bicycle (Figure 9-3c). As you complete your pedaling motion, straighten the leg behind you (Figure 9-3d) and swing it back forward to start the bicycling motion again.

After 3 forward pedals, reverse the pedaling by swinging your top leg back, bending it while the knee is still behind you, and extending the leg as it comes to the front. Do 3 backward pedals.

Do's and don'ts

- ✔ Do place your palm on the floor in front of you to help you maintain balance throughout the exercise, if you need to do so.

- ✔ Do keep your neck long and relaxed.

- ✔ Do keep your body square, hip over hip, and shoulder over shoulder.

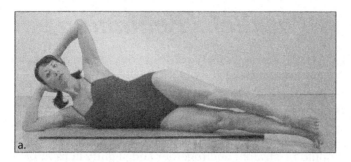

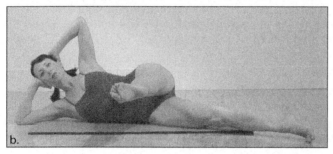

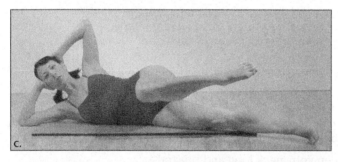

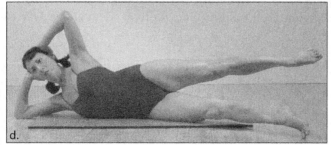

Figure 9-3:
Bicycle.

Up/Down in Parallel (Beginning)

Up/Down in Parallel strengthens the side of your hips and butt (the gluteus medius and gluteus minimus). You'll feel the burn!

Getting set

Lie on your side, propped up on one elbow with the hand supporting your head, and place your other arm's palm on the mat in front of you for support. Your legs should be straight and together and slightly in front of your body. Keep your hips square during the exercise. Point your knees straight ahead, in what is known as the parallel position. Point your feet. (Figure 9-4a shows the starting position.)

The exercise

Inhale: Lift your top leg about 1 foot off the floor (Figure 9-4b).

Exhale: Flex your foot at the top and bring your leg back down to the starting position, pulling your navel in and squeezing your butt.

Think of pressing down an imaginary spring as you lower your leg, creating resistance in the inner thigh. Imagine reaching your heel long away from you, as if your top leg will reach longer than your lower leg.

Complete 8 repetitions, alternating the pointing and flexing of the foot.

Do's and don'ts

✔ Do press your weight into the palm on the floor in front of you to maintain balance throughout the exercise.

✔ Do keep your neck long and relaxed.

✔ Do keep your body square, hip over hip and shoulder over shoulder.

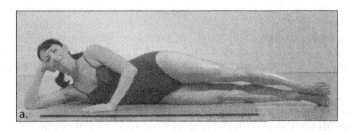

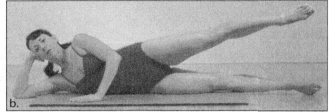

Figure 9-4:
Up/Down in
Parallel.

Butt Cruncher (Beginning)

Butt Cruncher addresses the side of the butt (the gluteus medius muscle) —
you know, the part you show if you wear a high-cut bikini. This exercise will
make you wince with pain, but it will give you the desired side-of-the-butt
firmness.

Getting set

Lie on your side propped up on one elbow, with the hand supporting your
head, and place your other arm's palm on the mat in front of you for support.
Fold your knees and hips at 90-degree angles and then straighten your top leg
so that it is at a 90-degree angle from your body. If you are tight in your legs,
come as close to 90 degrees as you can. You can also bend your knee slightly
to make this position more comfortable. Flex your top foot. (Figure 9-5a
shows the starting position.)

The exercise

This exercise has two parts: First you pulse and then you circle.

Pulses

Breathing continuously: Think of reaching your heel long away from you as
you lift and lower your top leg, making small pulsing movements (Figure 9-5b).
Accent the up direction of the movement for 8 pulses (think up and up and up
and up . . .).

Circles

Breathing continuously: Still reaching your heel long away from you, make small circles with your heel as if you're painting circles on the wall that's in front of you. Circle 8 times in one direction and then 8 times in the opposite direction.

Transition by straightening your lower leg, bending your top leg, and dropping your top knee down on the mat in front of your lower leg. Now you're ready for the Inner Thigh Pulses.

Do's and don'ts

- ✔ Do keep your body square, hip over hip and shoulder over shoulder.
- ✔ Don't let your leg turn in as you repeat the movements. Keep your knee facing straight ahead.

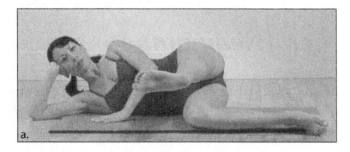

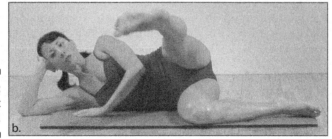

Figure 9-5:
Butt
Cruncher.

Inner Thigh Pulses (Beginning)

Women are always coming to me wanting to tone their inner thighs. Well, ladies, here's your exercise! Because this exercise works your inner thighs, it gives your butt a much-needed break.

Getting set

Lie on your side, one arm propping up your head and the other on the mat, and straighten out your lower leg. Bend your top leg and bring it in front of you so that your lower leg has room to move straight up (Figure 9-6a).

The exercise

Inhaling and exhaling: Flex your bottom foot and reach your heel long away from you as you lift and lower your leg, making large pulsing movements (Figure 9-6b). Try to lift your leg as high as you can without losing your control and balance. Think of initiating the movement from your belly by pulling your navel in toward your spine on every upward pulse.

Accent the up direction for 10 pulses — think up and up and up and up.

Transition to Up/Down in Turnout by straightening both legs and bringing them together, back to the side-lying position. Your legs should be slightly in front of your body. Place your top arm down on the mat for support.

Do's and don'ts

✔ Do lift your leg as high as you can, really challenging your inner thigh.

✔ Do keep your body square, hip over hip and shoulder over shoulder.

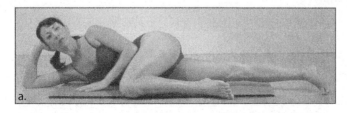

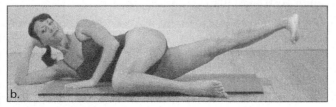

Figure 9-6:
Inner Thigh
Pulses.

Up/Down in Turnout (Beginning)

The model in this exercise is a ballet dancer and has incredible flexibility. Don't worry if you can't match her movements.

Up/Down in Turnout is so named because your legs are turned out, in contrast to the Up/Down in Parallel, in which your legs are both facing straight ahead.

Getting set

Lie on your side with your legs slightly in front of your body, turned out from the top of the hip, knees facing away from each other. Rest on one elbow, with the other hand on the mat in front of you for stability (Figure 9-7a). You can turn your bottom foot toward the floor to help stabilize the movement.

The exercise

Inhale: Kick your top leg straight up to the sky. Figure 9-7b shows the model kicking her leg *way* up to the sky. Don't feel that you need to go that high.

Exhale: Flex your foot, as shown in Figure 9-7c, at the top and bring your leg back down to the starting position. Pull your navel in and squeeze your butt as you lower your leg.

You're pressing down an imaginary spring as you lower your leg. Imagine that your top leg will reach longer than your lower leg as you stretch your heel away from you.

Complete 8 repetitions with each leg and then continue with Up/Down with Passé.

Do's and don'ts

✔ Do press your weight into the hand on the floor to maintain balance throughout the exercise.

✔ Do keep your neck long and relaxed.

✔ Do keep your body square, hip over hip and shoulder over shoulder.

✔ Don't let your leg bend as you lift it. Only go as high as you can while maintaining a straight leg.

✔ Don't let your leg turn in as you lift it; keep your knees facing away from each other as much as you can.

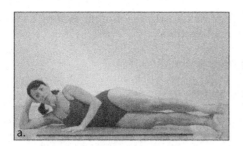

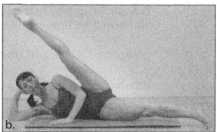

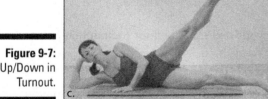

Figure 9-7:
Up/Down in
Turnout.

Up/Down with Passé (Intermediate)

Like in the previous exercise, keep in mind that the model is a ballet dancer and has incredible flexibility. Don't worry if you can't match her movements. Up/Down with Passé strengthens your hips, butt, and outer thighs while stretching the inner thighs.

Getting set

Lie on your side with your legs slightly in front of your body, turned out from the top of the hips, knees facing away from each other. Rest on one elbow, using your hand to support your head, and put your free palm on the mat in front of you for stability (Figure 9-8a). You can turn your bottom foot toward the floor to help stabilize the movement. Keep your feet pointed throughout this exercise.

The exercise

Inhale: Bend your top leg, bringing the knee up toward the ceiling (Figure 9-8b). Try to touch your pointed foot to the inside of the bottom knee (the passé position) and then straighten your leg up toward the sky (Figure 9-8c).

You are moving through honey, and there is a gooey resistance as you move your leg through space.

Exhale: Bring your straight leg back down, reaching it as long as you can as you bring the inner thighs back together.

Complete 4 times and then reverse the direction:

Inhale: Kick your top leg straight up to the sky.

Exhale: Bend your knee, trying to touch your foot to the inside of your bottom knee. Then straighten your top leg and bring the inner thighs back together.

Complete 4 times and then bring your legs together to do the Figure 8.

Do's and don'ts

- ✔ Do press your weight into your hand on the floor to maintain balance throughout the exercise.

- ✔ Do keep your neck long and relaxed.

- ✔ Do keep your body square, hip over hip and shoulder over shoulder.

- ✔ Don't let your leg bend as you lift it. Only go as high as you can while maintaining a straight leg.

- ✔ Don't let your leg turn in as you lift it; keep your knees facing away from each other as much as you can.

A new main squeeze

Here's a bonus exercise, Heel Squeezes, if you want even more butt and thigh work. You should do this exercise at the midpoint of your Side Kick series. In other words, once you've finished your series on one side, roll onto your belly and do the Heel Squeezes; then roll onto your other side to finish the series.

Lie flat on your belly with your forehead down on the mat, your hands underneath your forehead. Spread your legs apart, bend your knees, and bring your heels together. Your heels should be pointed straight up to the sky.

Breathing continuously: Press your heels together as you squeeze your butt and press your pubic bone down to the mat. Think of pulling your navel into your spine as you lift your belly up so that you could slide a piece of paper underneath your belly. Hold for 1 full breath and release. Complete 8 repetitions.

Heel Squeezes are a great way to tone your butt muscles. You should feel this exercise in your biggest butt muscle (the gluteus maximus).

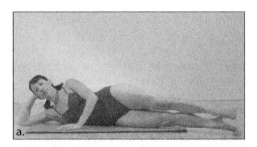

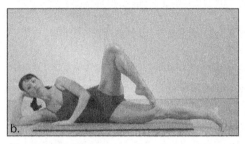

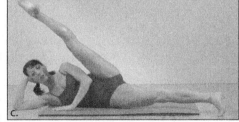

Figure 9-8:
Up/Down
with Passé.

Figure 8 (Intermediate)

This one can be harder on your brain than your butt. Getting the reverse
direction going can be a challenge, but it's a fun challenge. Figure 8 strengthens
the butt and inner thighs — and tones the concentration.

Getting set

The starting position for Figure 8 is the same as for Up/Down in Turnout and
Up/Down with Passé. Lie on your side with your legs slightly in front of your
body and slightly turned out in the Pilates First Position. Rest on one elbow
with the other hand on the mat in front of you for stability (Figure 9-9a). You
can turn your bottom foot toward the floor to help stabilize the movement.

The exercise

Breathing continuously: Lift your top leg slightly and begin drawing a figure 8 with your big toe. As you bring your leg to the back, squeeze your butt and use your Abdominal Scoop to maintain the stability in your body. Figures 9-9b and 9-9c show the figure 8 shape being made.

Complete 4 Figure 8s and then reverse the direction for 4 more. Bring your legs together for the pièce de résistance, Grande Ronde de Jambe!

Do's and don'ts

- ✔ Do press your weight into the hand on the floor to maintain balance throughout the exercise.

- ✔ Do feel your butt working each time you bring your leg to the back.

- ✔ Do keep your body square, hip over hip and shoulder over shoulder.

- ✔ Don't let your leg turn in as you repeat the figure 8s; keep turning your top knee slightly toward the ceiling.

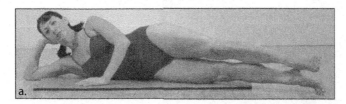

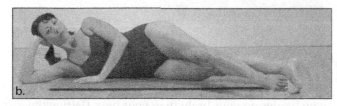

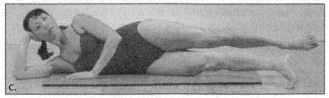

Figure 9-9:
Figure 8.

Grande Ronde de Jambe (Advanced)

Grande Ronde de Jambe (grrrond ron-day-jom) is French for "big circle of the leg." It sounds better in French, I think. It's a movement that's usually done in ballet (while standing), so that's why it has a French name.

This is by far my favorite butt-and-thigh exercise. You can really feel the burn when you're doing it right. The movement of the leg from the side to behind the body (or vice versa, when reversing directions) is the main movement that works your butt and saddlebags, so go through this part slowly in both directions and you'll feel the burn in the good places. Never jerk your leg up, or you'll be cheating your butt out of its much deserved exercise!

You should feel your butt as well as your outer thighs really working. The key is to go slowly through the hard parts. Find your butt and work it hard!

Getting set

Get into the same starting position you've used a number of times in this series, most recently for Figure 8. Lie on your side with your legs slightly in front of your body and turned out from the top of the hips, knees facing away from each other. Rest on one elbow, with the other hand on the mat in front of you for stability. You can turn your bottom foot toward the floor to help stabilize the movement.

The exercise

Inhale: Bring your top leg forward as far as you can, trying to maintain the turnout in your legs and the stability in your torso (Figure 9-10a).

Exhale: Continue moving your leg, circling it up to the side as close to your ear as you can. Squeeze your butt and use your Abdominal Scoop to maintain stability in your torso (Figure 9-10b).

Inhale: Finish with your leg behind you, but not more than 15 degrees behind your body. Figure 9-10c shows the leg going from as close to the ear as possible to behind the model. Continue to bring your leg down until it's level with your hips. Don't let your back arch as your leg goes behind you.

Imagine that someone is grabbing on to your ankle and pulling your leg away from your hip while you draw the biggest circle you can with your big toe.

Exhale: Bring your legs back together.

Complete 3 repetitions and reverse the direction of the circle for 3 more circles.

Do's and don'ts

- ✔ Do press your weight into the hand on the floor to maintain balance throughout the exercise.

- ✔ Do feel your butt working each time you bring your leg to the back.

- ✔ Do keep your body square, hip over hip and shoulder over shoulder.

- ✔ Don't let your leg turn in as you move your leg around in the circle. Keep turning your top knee toward the ceiling.

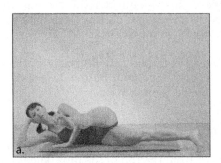
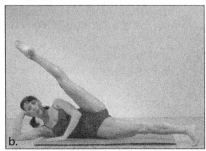
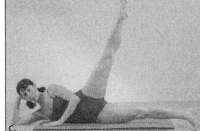

Figure 9-10:
Grande
Ronde de
Jambe.

Chapter 10

Meow! Stretching the Spine

. . . .

In This Chapter

▶ Performing simple and safe exercises to stretch out the back and get that kink out

▶ Seeing how Pilates uses cats as a model for a healthy spine

. . . .

*I*f you've ever watched a cat, be it a house cat or a jaguar, you may have been intrigued by the cat's incredible agility and resilience. How does a cat jump from high places and land with little impact? How can a cat fit into spaces that seem way too small for it? How does a cat balance on the slimmest edge with the greatest of ease? I don't know the answer to these questions, but I do know that if you want to be more like a cat and gain the flexibility, grace, balance, and strength of a cat, Pilates is the way to go.

Myth has it that Joe Pilates was obsessed with the movement of animals and used them as models when developing exercises. The following exercises use the cat as a model and are meant to stretch the spine. You may notice that the word *sexy* comes up in this chapter. Face it — having a flexible spine is sexy, and certain movements of the spine are downright sexy!

The exercises in this chapter are not considered part of classic Pilates, but they're great for everyone. They are all safe and fairly easy (Mermaid takes a little more finesse than the others). This is where you can get a little creative. Add in these exercises at any point during your day or during your workout when you feel you need to stretch out your spine. I like to do the Sexy Spine Stretch after a serious abdominal exercise because it gives my back a nice break and helps me continue with the workout. Find your favorite stretch and make it your own!

If you wake up in the morning with a stiff back or neck, spend a couple minutes doing one or two of the cat stretches.

All of the exercises that follow are considered beginning level, except for the Mermaid, which is intermediate.

Spine Stretches in This Chapter

Here's a preview of the stretches in this chapter:

- ✔ Basic Cat
- ✔ Hunting Cat
- ✔ Mermaid
- ✔ Sexy Spine Stretch

Basic Cat (Beginning)

The Basic Cat is one of the gentlest and simplest ways to stretch out the back. You see cats making this movement in the morning when they wake, and you can do it too!

Getting set

To begin, get on all fours. Align your hands beneath your shoulders and your knees beneath your hips. Allow your back to assume its natural position, in Neutral Spine (Figure 10-1a).

The exercise

Inhale: Arch your back slightly, allowing your head to rise and your butt to stick up and out (Figure 10-1b).

Exhale: Pull your navel in toward your spine and squeeze your low butt. You begin with a Lumbar C Curve, meaning that your lower back is curved like a C, then continue rounding into the upper back. Finally, allow the head to slowly drop forward. At this point, your whole spine should be making a C shape (Figure 10-1c). Your back should be rounded to the greatest extent possible.

Push your arms into the mat for extra resistance while stretching the upper back. Keep your abdominals and rib cage pulled in. Think of using this pulling action to stretch through your whole spine.

Think of pulling your tail between your legs and rounding your back into a Halloween kitty pose.

Inhale: Return to Neutral Spine, then go further into the arch, sticking your tail and head upward.

Complete 4 repetitions.

Sexy, sexy cat

The Sexy Cat is a modification of the Basic Cat and requires a bit more coordination. Because you spiral the hips and spine, this stretch is three-dimensional and loosens up more areas of tightness than the Basic Cat.

Start by doing one Basic Cat to get the flow of the spine arching and contracting. Then add a spiral in one direction with your hips, and in the opposite direction with your head and neck. Imagine the tailbone inscribing a full circle on the wall behind you in one direction, and the crown of your head inscribing a full circle on the wall in front of you in the other direction

Complete 4 repetitions and then reverse the direction of the spiral for 4 more repetitions.

Do's and don'ts

✔ Do go for the fullest stretch in each direction.

✔ Don't hunch your shoulders. Let them relax down away from your ears.

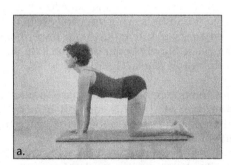

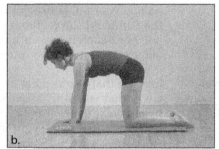

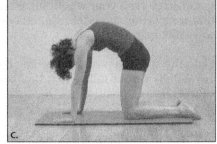

Figure 10-1: Basic Cat.

Hunting Cat (Beginning)

The Hunting Cat was developed by Kathy Grant, who was one of Joe Pilates' original students. She's still teaching in Manhattan. She loves cats and has developed several variations of the Basic Cat exercise (including the Sexy Cat). This is but one of many such variations. This variation teaches you how to articulate your lumbar spine (lower back) independently of your thoracic spine (upper back), which is not as easy as it sounds.

Watch yourself do this exercise head-on in a mirror. You should not see any movement of the spine until you're ready to pounce.

Getting set

Get on all fours. Align your hands beneath your shoulders and your knees beneath your hips. Allow your back to assume its natural position, in Neutral Spine (Figure 10-2a). Take a deep breath in.

The exercise

Exhale: As shown in Figure 10-2b, begin by rounding your low back. Think of pulling your tail between your legs and hollowing your lowest belly to begin the Lumbar C Curve. Remember to try to move only your lower back at first, and not hunch into your upper back. Slowly begin to sit back on your heels, allowing the stretch to round the whole back (Figure 10-2c).

Imagine that you're a cat about to pounce on prey. Prepare to pounce in such a way that you don't alarm your poor victim This can only be accomplished by moving the lower back independently of the upper back. Once the upper back starts to round, your imaginary prey will see you moving!

Inhale: Once you're all the way back on your heels, slowly pounce forward like a Halloween kitty, rounding and stretching your whole spine and coming as far forward as you can on your arms (your shoulders should come in front of your hands). Figure 10-2d shows this position.

Exhale: Lead with your tail back to the starting position, coming back to Neutral Spine. Imagine someone pulling on your tail so that the base of your spine brings you back to the neutral starting position.

Complete 4 repetitions.

Do's and don'ts

✔ Do pull your belly in to increase the stretch into your back.

✔ Do watch yourself in a mirror, if you can.

✔ Don't let your shoulders hunch up by your ears.

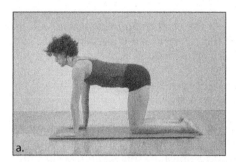
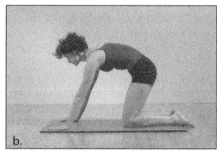
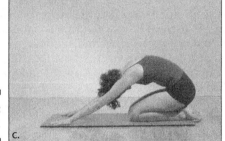
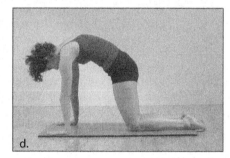

Figure 10-2: Hunting Cat.

Mermaid (Intermediate)

You can do the Mermaid exercise on the mat and on all the pieces of Pilates equipment. It is an excellent stretch for the sides of the torso (both the side abdominal and the side back muscles). I recommend it for people with lower back tightness and chest tightness. You'll know if you have tightness in these areas once you try this exercise! It feels wonderful.

Getting set

Sit on your left hip, with your knees bent and your legs folded on top of each other, feet facing toward the right and behind you. You can adjust the legs to be either on top of one another or more separate until you find a comfortable position for your hips. You should be sitting like a mermaid, with your tail to one side. Figure 10-3a shows the mermaid position.

You can sit on a pillow if your knees hurt in the initial position, or you can straighten out the top leg to the side.

The exercise

Inhale: Place your left elbow down on the mat beside you. Simultaneously, reach the right arm overhead as far as you can (Figure 10-3b).

Exhale: Reverse the direction of the stretch and reach your left arm overhead, thinking of pulling your navel in toward your spine or using your Abdominal Scoop (Figure 10-3c). This is your side stretch position.

Inhale: Repeat the first movement by putting your left elbow down by your side and reaching your right arm overhead.

Breathing continuously: Reverse the direction of the stretch and reach your left arm overhead, thinking of pulling your navel in toward your spine or using your Abdominal Scoop. Now add a spiral to this stretch by arching your back and reaching your arm as far back as you can (Figure 10-3d). I call this part carving the sphere. Continue the stretch by making the biggest circle you can with your arm. As your arm comes in front of you, your back should now round forward (Figure 10-3e). Pulling your navel in and scooping your belly, complete the circle and come back to the side stretch position. Reverse the circle of your arm, rounding your back as you circle forward and arching your back as your arm circles behind you.

Imagine that someone is holding your hand and pulling your arm in the biggest possible circle it can make.

Do only once and repeat the exercise on the other side.

Do's and don'ts

✔ Do allow your arm to reach far back behind your body to open your chest and give you the maximum chest stretch.

✔ Do sit on a pillow if your knees hurt.

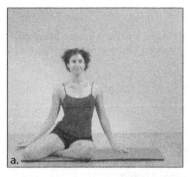
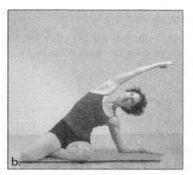
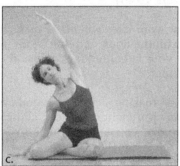
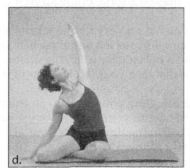
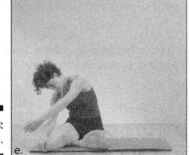

Figure 10-3: Mermaid.

Sexy Spine Stretch (Beginning)

This exercise was named by an 8-year-old girl that I used to teach dance to. She called it sexy because the position that you end up in is somewhat luxurious and looks a little like a *Playboy* cover. Again, it's an excellent stretch for the spine and the chest.

This stretch involves twisting the spine, which is not a good movement if you have a bulging intervertebral disc injury. If you have been diagnosed with this condition, please proceed with caution. If this exercise creates an uncomfortable sensation in your spine, please don't do it.

Getting set

Lie on your back with your left leg straight in the air, the knee bent at a 90-degree angle, and your right leg straight on the mat in front of you (see Figure 10-4a).

The exercise

Inhale: Breathe in deeply.

Exhale: Cross your left leg over your body until your knee makes contact with the floor. Grab the left knee with your right hand to keep it steady and to increase the force of the stretch (Figure 10-4b).

If you have a very tight back or chest, your knee will never make it to the floor and your left shoulder will pop off the floor, and that's fine. You want to find a balance between the distance your left shoulder comes off the mat and the distance your left knee is off the mat.

Inhale: Drag your left arm on the floor, making a circle that ends with your arm next to your left ear. As your arm approaches your ear, allow your body to roll in the direction of your arm so that you end up lying on your side with your arm by your ear (Figure 10-4c).

Exhale: Drag your left arm in the opposite direction and allow yourself to roll back onto your back, again dragging your arm heavy on the floor to maximize the chest stretch.

You can lie in the ending position, with your left arm making a T with your body and your right arm holding the left leg. Breathe deeply and feel the stretch deepen as you lie there.

Do only once and repeat the exercise on the other side.

Rock out (your back), man

Rocking out your back is a great exercise to do anytime your back is tired or stiff from doing really difficult abdominal exercises. Lying on your back, bring your knees into your chest. Place one hand on each knee. Make gentle circles with your tucked-in legs, allowing your back to get a massage on the mat beneath you. After 3 circles, reverse directions.

Do's and don'ts

✔ Do keep your arm heavy on the floor as you drag it to open the chest to give you the maximal chest stretch.

✔ Don't continue if your low back feels compressed or pinched or if you feel shooting pain.

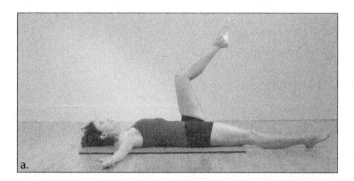

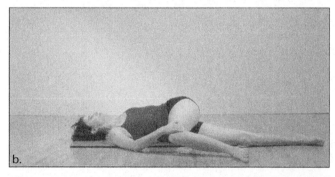

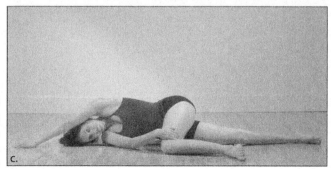

Figure 10-4:
Sexy Spine
Stretch.

Part III

Beyond the Mat: Exercises Using Equipment and Accessories

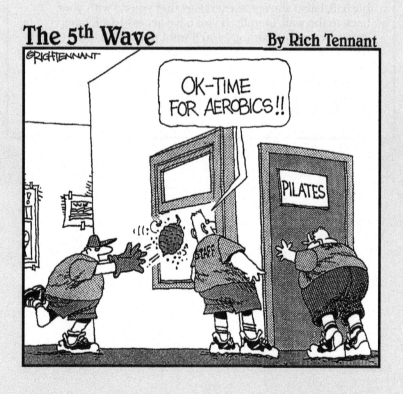

The 5th Wave By Rich Tennant

OK-TIME FOR AEROBICS!!

PILATES

Part III

Beyond the Mat: Exercises Using Equipment and

In this part . . .

You can enhance your Pilates routine by using equipment. In this part, I show you how to use neat pieces of small equipment, including the roller, the small ball, and the big ball. I also show you exercises that you do with your back to the wall, literally. If you have access to a Pilates studio or are just curious, you'll want to read Chapter 15, in which I discuss the heavy equipment of Pilates.

All you need to have a great Pilates experience is a mat. But if you want to ratchet your Pilates up a notch and introduce some more variety, read on!

Chapter 11

Plastic Foam Never Felt So Good: The Roller

*T*he roller is one of the most addictive accessories at my studio. You'll be surprised at how effective a cylinder of plastic foam can be. (Flip forward a few pages for a glimpse of the roller in action.)

In my Pilates studio, my staff and I use the roller to help people stretch out their chest muscles (pectorals) and to realign their neck and upper back. Using the roller is one of the best ways to alleviate upper back and neck pain. We also use the roller to massage many of the muscles of the body. You can do hundreds of things with the roller; in this chapter I mention just a few of my favorites. If you want more exercises, books are available through OPTP, a supplier for rehabilitation specialists (www.optp.com). OPTP also sells rollers.

If you feel like it's too difficult to stay on the roller without tensing up your body, then you're not ready to do these exercises. Try doing them on the mat instead. After you've mastered them on the mat, go back on the roller.

Do all the exercises listed here in the order shown; they're meant to be done one after another. All the roller exercises described in this chapter except the Swan start in the same position and are meant to flow from one to the next.

Originally, practitioners of the Feldenkreis method used the roller, so rollers are sometimes called Feldenkreis rollers. Feldenkreis is also called "awareness through movement," and it's another movement system to help people feel aligned and more in touch with their bodies. Even though the roller isn't a part of classic Pilates, it's a wonderful tool to use in conjunction with Pilates exercises because it helps people better feel the alignment and posture they're striving for.

Note: All the exercises in this chapter are considered beginning level.

Exercises in This Chapter

The exercises in this chapter are divided into the basic shoulder set and other roller exercises. The basic shoulder set was developed by yours truly to open up and stretch the chest muscles (pectorals), teach proper neck and shoulder alignment, and release the upper back and neck. The basic shoulder set is an excellent way to start your mat workout, because once you're opened up in this way, it is easier to incorporate Pilates mat concepts and to find proper alignment in your spine.

Basic shoulder set

✓ Shoulder Slaps

✓ Arm Reaches/Arm Circles

✓ Chicken Wings

✓ Angels in the Snow

Other roller exercises

✓ Tiny Steps

✓ The Swan

Shoulder Slaps

I describe how to do Shoulder Slaps as a mat exercise in Chapter 4. When you do them on the roller, Shoulder Slaps are even more effective at releasing your shoulder muscles and teaching proper shoulder placement.

Getting set

To get into the starting position, sit on the edge of the roller and roll slowly down onto your back, placing your hands on the floor to help you control the movement down. Now you should be lying back with the roller along your spine, your knees bent, your feet flat on the floor approximately hip distance apart, your arms down by your sides, and your palms facing down. Make sure that your head and your whole spine are on the roller; adjust forward or back if you're falling off. The roller is too unstable for you to maintain Neutral Spine; instead, flatten your low back onto the roller by using your Abdominal Scoop. (Neutral Spine and Abdominal Scoop are parts of the Pilates alphabet. See Chapter 3 for more information.)

The exercise

Inhale: Reach your arms up to the sky, allowing your scapulae (shoulder blades) to come off the roller (Figure 11-1a).

Exhale: Keep your arms straight as you completely relax and release the shoulder muscles, letting your scapulae slap back down (Figure 11-1b).

Complete 4 repetitions. On the final repetition, allow your scapulae to come down slowly, imagining your shoulder blades melting down into the back. Keep pushing your scapulae back and feel the muscles that are working. This concept of having "your shoulders down your back" is very important and is repeated over and over again in Pilates.

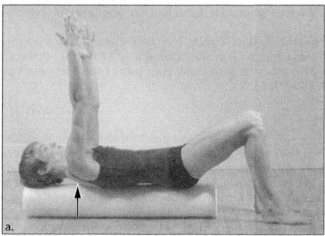

Lift your shoulders off the roller…

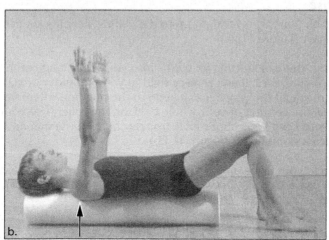

Figure 11-1:
Shoulder
Slaps.

and then let them slap back down.

Do's and don'ts

✔ Do really release on the exhale, allowing your shoulder blades and arms to truly drop with gravity.

✔ Don't bend your arms when you slap your shoulder blades down.

Arm Reaches/Arm Circles

You can do Arm Reaches/Arm Circles (which I describe in Chapter 4) on the mat as well as on the roller. Like Shoulder Shrugs, this exercise is even more effective in both its goals — stretching out your chest and back muscles and teaching upper torso stability — when done on the roller. Feel free to hold the stretch if it feels good and if you feel like you need it.

If you're tight and need to stretch, focus on opening your chest when performing this exercise. If you're a noodle and have lots of flexibility in your body, then focus on stabilizing your torso (don't let your upper back arch off the roller!).

Getting set

You should already be in the correct position after doing Shoulder Slaps. The roller is along your spine, your knees are bent, your feet are flat on the floor approximately hip distance apart, your arms are down by your sides, and your palms are facing down. Make sure that your head and your whole spine are on the roller; adjust forward or back if you're falling off the edge. The roller is too unstable for you to maintain Neutral Spine; instead, flatten your lower back onto the roller by using your Abdominal Scoop.

The exercise

Inhale: Reach your arms straight up to the ceiling, keeping them shoulder distance apart (Figure 11-2a).

Exhale: First, think of knitting your ribs into your belly, and reach your arms back toward your ears. If you're very tight in your shoulder area, you may not be able to reach all the way back. Just go to the position where you feel a stretch. Feel the contact of your whole back on the roller; use your upper abdominals to keep your upper back from arching off the mat and to keep your ribs from popping up (Figure 11-2b).

Inhale: Circle your arms open to a T shape (keeping the arms heavy on the floor) then down by your sides, then back to the starting position, reaching up to the sky.

Complete 3 repetitions and reverse directions.

On the last circle, allow your arms to reach all the way back by your ears, trying to keep your arms on the floor. Allow your back to arch and your chest to expand open. Take a deep breath in and expand into your rib cage and lungs. This movement will transition you into the next exercise, Chicken Wings.

Do's and don'ts

✔ Do maintain absolute stability in your torso by keeping your ribs down until the very last repetition.

✔ Do keep your shoulders down away from your ears as you initiate the exercise.

✔ Don't let your upper back arch off the roller until the end. This is the whole point of this exercise! As you raise your arms, your upper back naturally wants to go with them. Figure 11-3 shows the back arched off the mat. This is a model of what *not* to do . . . until the last one, when you can go for your stretch.

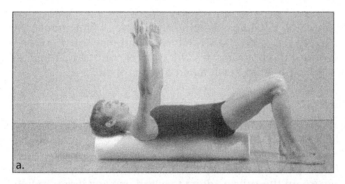

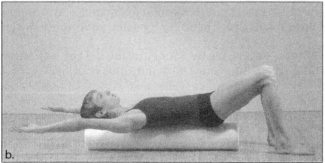

Figure 11-2:
Arm
Reaches/
Arm Circles.

Keep your back on the roller.

Figure 11-3:
How *not* to
do Arm
Reaches/
Arm Circles.

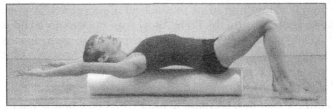

Don't allow your back to arch off the roller.

Chicken Wings

If you were a chicken, your shoulder blades would be your wings, right? In this exercise, you imagine that you're pulling your shoulder blades down your back so you're getting in touch with your inner chicken. The name *Chicken Wings* comes from one of my first Pilates teachers from San Francisco, Jennifer Stacey, an extremely knowledgeable woman. I believe she created this exercise.

Chicken Wings is a delicious stretch for your chest and shoulder muscles. If you're extremely tight and the stretch is too intense for whatever reason, roll off the roller onto the floor and try the exercise on the mat instead. As your muscles begin to open up, try it again on the roller.

Getting set

You should already be in the correct position after doing Arm Reaches/Arm Circles. The roller is along your spine, your knees are bent, your feet are flat on the floor approximately hip distance apart, your arms are down by your sides, and your palms are facing down. Make sure that your head and your whole spine are on the roller; adjust forward or back if you're falling off the edge. The roller is too unstable for you to maintain Neutral Spine; instead, flatten your lower back onto the roller by using your Abdominal Scoop.

Inhale: Reach your arms back by your ears, toward the wall behind you (Figure 11-4a). Expand into your chest and allow your back to arch off the roller a little.

Exhale: Start to slowly bend your elbows, trying to let them touch the floor as you pull them down, as if aiming them for your back pockets (Figure 11-4b). If you're very tight, your elbows won't touch the floor, so just let them drop back as far as feels comfortable. Try to keep your upper arm and lower arm at about a 90-degree angle to each other as you do the exercise. Imagine pulling your shoulder blades down your back with your back muscles. Once you've pulled your elbows down as far as you can, let your arms straighten and come down by your sides.

Inhale: Turn your palms up to the sky and go right into Angels in the Snow.

Complete 3 repetitions alternating Chicken Wings and Angels in the Snow.

Do's and don'ts

- ✔ Do allow your arms to drop down to the mat to get your best stretch.
- ✔ Do allow your back to arch off the roller to get a better stretch in your chest.
- ✔ Do inhale deeply and hold any part of the movement that feels like a particularly great stretch.

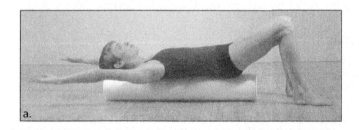

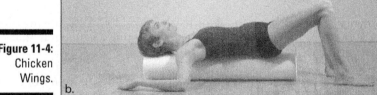

Figure 11-4:
Chicken
Wings.

Angels in the Snow

When I was a kid growing up in Philly, we used to get so excited when it snowed and we could run outside and make snow angels. Even though I've lived in California for over 15 years, I still like to make snow angels in my mind. Angels in the Snow is a great exercise for teaching the proper shoulder alignment while stretching out the chest (the pectoral muscles).

Getting set

You should already be in the correct position after doing Chicken Wings. The roller is along your spine, your knees are bent, your feet are flat on the floor approximately hip distance apart, your arms are down by your sides, and your palms are facing up. Make sure that your head and your whole spine are on the roller; adjust forward or back if you're falling off the edge. The roller is too unstable for you to maintain Neutral Spine; instead, flatten your lower back onto the roller by using your Abdominal Scoop. Take a deep breath in.

The exercise

Exhale: Pull your shoulder blades down your back as you begin to drag your arms slowly along the floor, opening them to a T shape with your body (Figure 11-5a).

You're making angels in the snow with your arms. Imagine that you're lying in the snow and pushing up the snow with your arms by using your back muscles and allowing your chest to open and release.

Inhale: Keep your arms heavy on the floor to get a wonderful stretch in your chest as you allow your arms to keep moving, completing a semicircle that ends with your arms up by your ears (Figure 11-5b).

Exhale: Move your arms back down with the Chicken Wings motion from the previous exercise: Slowly bend your elbows, trying to let them touch the floor as you pull them down, as if aiming them for your back pockets. If you're very tight, your elbows won't touch the floor, so just let them drop back as far as feels comfortable. Try to keep your upper arms and lower arms at about a 90-degree angle to each other as you do the exercise. Imagine pulling your shoulder blades down your back with your back muscles. Once you've pulled your elbows down as far as you can, let your arms straighten and come down by your sides.

Alternate Angels in the Snow (going up with your arms) and Chicken Wings (coming down with your arms).

Complete 3 repetitions.

Do's and don'ts

✔ Do allow your arms to stay heavy on the floor, and try to drag them only from the back muscles.

✔ Do inhale deeply and hold any part of the movement that feels like a particularly great stretch.

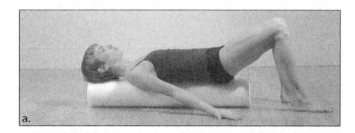

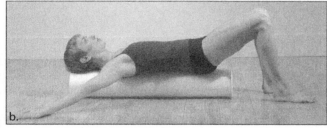

Figure 11-5:
Angels in
the Snow.

Tiny Steps

Any mat stability exercise becomes more challenging when you do it on the roller, and Tiny Steps is no exception. I describe Tiny Steps in Chapter 4 as a mat exercise, and it's hard enough on the mat. But on the roller, it's a killer. You see, the roller likes to wobble from side to side; that's what round things like to do. To keep the roller from rolling, you must engage even deeper into your core muscles.

Tiny Steps is a stability exercise that tests the strength and stability of your lower abdominals. The point of this exercise is to not move your hips or lower back while moving your legs up and down. It looks simple, but it actually takes quite a bit of inner strength. You're going for absolute stability here!

Feel free to use your arms pressing on the floor to help you stabilize yourself during this exercise, and make sure that your whole back makes contact with the roller (Figure 11-6a).

Getting set

You should already be in the correct position after doing Angels in the Snow. The roller is along your spine, your knees are bent, your feet are flat on the floor approximately hip distance apart, your arms are down by your sides, and your palms are facing down. Make sure that your head and your whole spine are on the roller; adjust forward or back if you're falling off the edge. The roller is too unstable for you to maintain Neutral Spine; instead, flatten your lower back onto the roller by using your Abdominal Scoop. Take a deep breath in.

Exhale: Pull your navel in toward your spine and lift your right knee up to your chest (Figure 11-6b).

Inhale: Maintain the position.

Exhale: Bring your right leg back down to the mat, controlling the movement from the center, and return to the starting position.

Alternate sides and repeat 8 times.

Do's and don'ts

- Don't let your lower back arch or your hips rock side to side.
- Don't tense your upper body when doing this exercise. Keep your neck long and your shoulders relaxed.

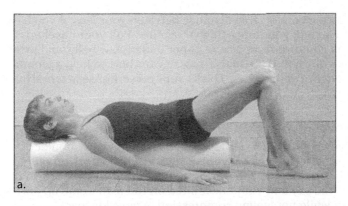

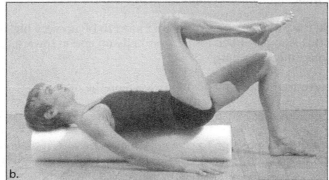

Figure 11-6:
Tiny Steps.

The Swan

The Swan is a basic back extension exercise. A version called Rising Swan is in Chapter 5, and a super advanced version called Swan Dive is in Chapter 8. The Swan on the roller is a gentle way to discover how to extend your spine and mostly shows you proper neck and shoulder alignment. The exercise also strengthens the muscles of the neck and upper back, which is very important to correct slouching posture and rounded shoulders.

Getting set

Lie on your belly with your forehead flat on the mat and your arms up on the roller in front of you. Position your arms so that your wrists make contact with the roller, and turn your palms toward each other in a karate chop position. Your arms should be a little wider than shoulder width apart. Allow your legs to turn out from the top of your hip (in other words, drop your heels toward each other). See Figure 11-7a.

You can keep a comfortable distance between your legs; if you have slim hips, you can pull your inner thighs together. Pull your navel up off the mat so that you could slide a piece of paper under your belly, and press your pubic bone down into the mat. Squeeze your butt to help accomplish this tucking under of your pelvis. This is your powerhouse at work! Inhale deeply to begin.

The exercise

Exhale: Slowly pull the roller toward you, sliding your shoulder blades down your back as you slowly raise your head and neck up off the floor (Figure 11-7b). Come up into the Swan position with your crown reaching up toward the sky and your chest lifted off the mat. Come up only as high as you can while not feeling compression in your low back.

Inhale: Hold the Swan position. You don't need to be up very high to get the benefits of this exercise. Keep lifting your belly up and in toward the spine and keep squeezing your butt.

Exhale: Return to the starting position, down on the mat.

Complete 3 repetitions.

Push back to the rest position to give your back a break (sit on your heels so that you're rounded and relaxed forward in your spine like a fetus).

Do's and don'ts

- ✔ Do support your head by keeping your neck long and strong.
- ✔ Don't allow your lower back to sag; keep your powerhouse working overtime.

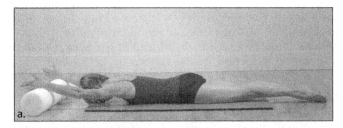

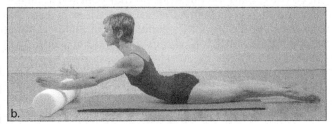

Figure 11-7:
The Swan.

Chapter 12

Abracadabra! The Magic Circle or a Small Ball

In This Chapter

▶ Knowing the difference between the circle and the ball

▶ Realizing the benefits of using the circle or the ball

*T*he magic circle is a classic piece of Pilates equipment. It basically consists of a metal ring with two cushions on either side for comfort when squeezing. In my studio, the magic circle is mostly used between the knees or ankles to work the inner thigh muscles. You also can hold it in your hands and push it to work the chest (the pectoral muscles). Pilates teachers around the world have developed hundreds of different variations of exercises that use the magic circle.

Honestly, I usually replace the magic circle with a simple rubber or plastic ball. The photos in this chapter all show the exercises being done with a small ball. A ball is much cheaper than a magic circle, and my studio has lots of group Pilates classes — using balls is simply easier. Also, the magic circle can pop out from between your ankles and knees, so it requires a bit more coordination just to keep it in place. The magic circle tends to be a little less comfortable to squeeze than a ball, and many magic circles are fairly difficult to squeeze, as compared to a soft and supple ball.

Maybe I'm biased, but I think that a simple ball approximately 6 to 8 inches in diameter and of medium softness is the perfect accessory for Pilates mat exercises. In my studio, I prefer the Gertie Ball (a brand name), a very nice small ball that you blow up with a straw.

Don't use a sports ball like a basketball or soccer ball. The main quality you're looking for in a ball is elasticity. You want it to rebound after you squeeze it. An elastic ball makes you use your muscles and won't give you bruises if you squeeze too hard. You should be able to find a good ball at a big drugstore or toy store. It doesn't need to be any special anything, just the right size and not too hard.

If you'd rather try a magic circle, you can purchase one from any Pilates equipment manufacturer (search the Web). Magic circles may have different names, depending on where you're buying them, but usually the word "circle" will be in it.

Almost all of these exercises are in previous chapters without a ball. If you have a ball, simply do the following exercises in the order that they are normally listed in the series in Chapters 4 through 7. Deep Abdominal Cue is the only exercise which is especially designed for the ball, and this one you want to do right before Upper Abdominal Curls.

Exercises in This Chapter

Here are the exercises in this chapter:

- Deep Abdominal Cue
- Upper Abdominal Curls
- Bridge
- Rollover
- Open Leg Rocker
- Around the World (Advanced)

Deep Abdominal Cue (Fundamental)

Deep Abdominal Cue is so easy that I don't even include photographs. Yet, it's so hard that the concept it teaches may elude you!

Here goes: Engaging the inner thigh muscles when doing an abdominal exercise helps you to find the deep abdominal muscles. The inner thigh muscles and the deep abdominal muscles work together, so when you use one it's easier to use the other. Every time you have the ball between your knees when doing an exercise, you can feel this deep abdominal connection.

Don't worry if you don't quite get the Deep Abdominal Cue. You'll still be fine with the rest of the exercises if you can't quite feel what I describe.

Getting set

Lie down on your back with your knees bent and your feet flat on the floor, about hip distance apart. Relax your back into Neutral Spine. Place the small ball between your knees. Place your hands on either side of your low belly, resting your fingers right inside the hip bones. Your hands are here to feel the deep abdominal muscles working. Take a deep breath in.

The exercise

Exhale: Pull the navel in toward the spine and slowly squeeze the ball, imagining that you are initiating the squeeze from the muscles right inside the hip bones (these are your abdominal obliques). Think of pulling your hip bones toward each other from these muscles underneath your fingers. Try to make these muscles harden as you squeeze the ball.

Inhale: Slowly loosen your grip on the ball and relax your belly.

Slowly complete 4 repetitions. Go right into your Upper Abdominal Curls.

Do's and don'ts

- ✔ Do think while you do this exercise. Really try and feel those connections between the muscles of your body.

- ✔ Don't let your lower back flatten. Instead, keep the tailbone anchored to the mat. Maintain Neutral Spine.

Upper Abdominal Curls (Fundamental)

I introduce Upper Abdominal Curls as a fundamental mat exercise in Chapter 4. I always teach this exercise to new clients in their first session, and I always use the ball when I teach it. Using the ball allows you to engage your inner thigh muscles and keeps your legs in proper alignment. As you hopefully will experience, the small ball also helps you feel your deep abdominal muscles.

Make sure that you first do the Deep Abdominal Cue before doing this exercise.

Lie down on your back with your knees bent and your feet flat on the floor, about hip distance apart. Relax your back into Neutral Spine. Place the small ball or magic circle between your knees. Interlace your fingers and put your hands behind your head. (See Figure 12-1a.)

The exercise

Exhale: Pull your navel in toward your spine, gently squeeze the ball (using your deep abdominal muscles to help) and lift your head, pulling your chin in toward your chest. As you lift your head, think of squeezing a tangerine under your chin as you roll up to your Pilates Abdominal Position; your head should be just high enough that your shoulder blades are barely off the mat (Figure 12-1b).

Inhale: Control the movement back down to the mat as you slowly release the squeeze on your ball.

Slowly complete 8 repetitions.

Do's and don'ts

> ✔ Do maintain Neutral Spine as you roll up.
>
> ✔ Don't let your lower back flatten, but keep your tailbone anchored to the mat.
>
> ✔ Don't strain your neck — allow your hands to hold the weight of your head and keep the space of a tangerine between your chin and your neck.

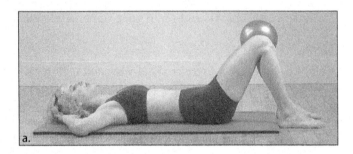

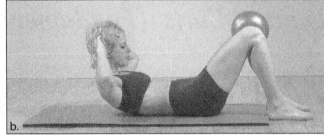

Figure 12-1: Upper Abdominal Curls.

Bridge (Beginning)

The Bridge exercise was first presented in the beginning series in Chapter 5. It's an excellent exercise to strengthen your butt and the back of your legs and to teach core stability. Adding the magic circle or ball between your knees brings in your inner thigh muscles and keeps proper alignment of your legs.

Getting set

Lie on your back with your knees bent and your feet flat on the floor, approximately hip distance apart. Your feet should be in a comfortable position, not too close to your butt and not too far away. You should be able to easily find the Neutral Spine. Experiment with different placements of your feet to find the best fit. Place your arms by your sides, palms down. (See Figure 12-2a.)

Put the magic circle or ball between your knees. Make sure that you squeeze it enough to keep your hips, knees, and feet in line. If the ball is bigger than 8 inches in diameter, your knees may be wider than your feet and hips, so if you have to, open your feet a little wider to accommodate the ball. Take a deep breath in.

The exercise

Exhale: Press your feet into the mat and squeeze your butt as you lift your hips up off the mat. Your body should make a straight line from your shoulders to your knees. Don't press up so high that you can't see your knees (Figure 12-2b).

Inhale: Hold the Bridge position.

Exhale: Think of knitting your ribs down to your belly, squeeze your butt, and try to lengthen through the front of your hips.

Inhale: Arch your spine up by lifting your hips higher, and think of inflating your back up like a balloon.

Exhale: Roll slowly down your spine one vertebra at a time. Use the Abdominal Scoop to press your lower back onto the mat as you come back to Neutral Spine.

Complete 5 repetitions.

Transition by bringing your knees into your chest to relax your back.

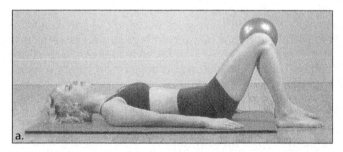

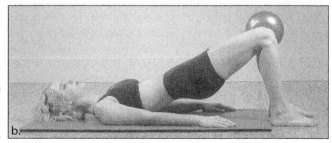

Figure 12-2:
Bridge.

Do's and don'ts

✔ Do maintain a plank position when up in the Bridge. Try not to arch your back.

✔ Do attempt to articulate through your spine on the way down.

✔ Do minimize the tension in your upper body; keep your neck long and relaxed.

Rollover (Advanced)

The Rollover was first presented as an advanced exercise in Chapter 7. With the addition of the ball between your ankles, you can really work your inner thighs and better find your deep Abdominal Scoop. This exercise demands a great amount of core strength, but when accomplished, it's a great stretch for your back and neck muscles. Try the classic Rollover first, without the ball, and then try this variation.

If you have lower back or neck problems, avoid this exercise.

Getting set

Lie flat on your back with your arms down by your sides, your palms facing down, and your legs straight up to the sky with a small ball or magic circle between your ankles (Figure 12-3a).

The exercise

Inhale: Pull your belly in, squeeze your butt and the ball or magic circle, and lift your legs up and over your head. Your legs should stop once they're parallel to the floor behind you. Don't let your toes touch the floor behind you. Don't roll onto your neck; stop and balance on your shoulders instead.

Exhale: Flex your feet, as shown in Figure 12-3b, and slowly roll back down your spine (Figure 12-3c). Press your palms and arms down on the floor to help you control the movement. Once your tailbone has touched down, allow your legs to continue to drop down toward the floor in front of you, but don't drop them so low that you can't maintain a flattened lower back (Figure 12-3d). Use your Abdominal Scoop and your butt squeeze to help you keep your lower back flat on the mat. Don't let your lower back arch off the mat even a little!

Inhale: Squeeze your ball or magic circle and begin the sequence again.

Complete 4 repetitions.

End by bending your knees into your chest and releasing your back.

Do's and don'ts

> ✔ Do keep the movement flowing and controlled.

> ✔ Don't roll up onto your neck. Think of keeping your neck long.

Modifications

To make this exercise easier, when you return from the Rollover, bring your legs back to this 90-degree angle and practice lowering your legs little by little every time you repeat the exercise. Don't lower your legs so low that you can't keep a flattened lower back on the mat. If your lower back arches off *at all* as you lower your legs, stop and bring your legs back up again. Doing so will protect your lower back. As you gain more abdominal strength, you'll be able to lower your legs more and more until you can start with them on the floor.

If your back is tight and you'd like to get more stretch out of this exercise, start the first Rollover and stop at the top, with your legs overhead, and grab onto each calf with your hands. Roll slowly down your spine, using your arms to help you stretch into your back. Then continue with the sequence.

If you're feeling up for a challenge, try the Rollover-Teaser combo! Start the basic Rollover, first lifting your legs up and over your head. As you roll down your spine and your tailbone hits the mat, allow your legs to drop to a 45-degree angle to the floor, and then roll up into the Teaser position, reaching your arms up in front of you. Then roll back down your spine and begin your next Rollover. Repeat 4 times and, on the last one, at the top of your Teaser, grab onto your ankles or calves and do the Open Leg Rocker. Figure 12-4 shows the Teaser variation.

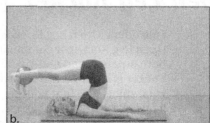
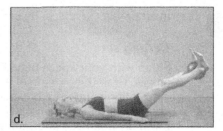
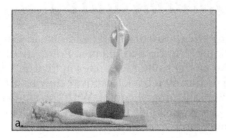
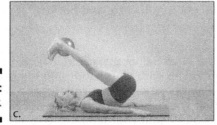

Figure 12-3:
Rollover.

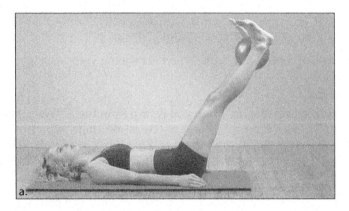

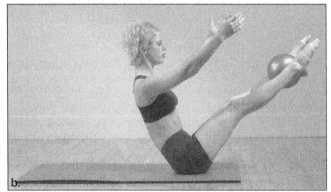

Figure 12-4:
The Teaser
modification
of the
Rollover.

Open Leg Rocker (Intermediate)

I introduce Open Leg Rocker as an intermediate mat exercise in Chapter 6.
Open Leg Rocker, a combination of Hip-Up and Balance Point, incorporates
both strength and control. Like all the rolling exercises in Pilates, Open Leg
Rocker is a fun way to massage your own back, discover how to articulate
your spine, and find your abdominal control center. With the small ball or
magic circle between your ankles, your inner thighs start kicking in, and your
deep Abdominal Scoop becomes more accessible.

In all rolling exercises, be careful not to roll onto your neck!

Getting set

Sit up with your knees bent and a small ball or magic circle between your
ankles. Grab the outside of your ankles with your hands and roll back behind
your tailbone into the Balance Point position, lifting your legs up off the mat
and straightening them up so that your legs and body make a V. Keep your
low belly hollowed and remain a bit behind your tailbone to feel the
Abdominal Scoop helping you balance.

If you have tight hamstrings (the muscles on the back of your legs) or a tight back, hold your legs closer to your knees instead of your ankles and try bending your legs slightly. (See Figure 12-5a.)

The exercise

Inhale: Roll back onto your upper back and do a Hip-Up, using your lower Abdominal Scoop to lift your hips. Squeeze your butt to get an extra lift. Your legs are now above you, parallel to the floor (Figure 12-5b).

Exhale: Return to your Balance Point, using your Abdominal Scoop as the brake to the rolling.

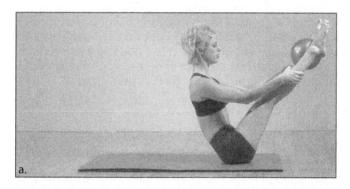

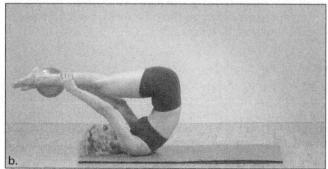

Figure 12-5:
Open Leg
Rocker.

Do's and don'ts

- ✔ Do think of massaging your back by hollowing out your abdominals to help you articulate each vertebra.
- ✔ Do allow your momentum to help you roll backward, and control the movement with your abdominals at the top of the Hip-Up.

> ✔ Do come back to your Balance Point, using your abdominals to find the control in the movement and to put the brakes on the momentum.
>
> ✔ Don't allow your back to make a thumping sound, especially on the way back up. Use your abdominals to pull into your lower back to make a smooth movement.

Around the World (Advanced)

Around the World is a lot like the Super Advanced Corkscrew in Chapter 8. Having the small ball or magic circle between your ankles works the inner thigh muscles and helps you find your deep Abdominal Scoop. Like the Super Advanced Corkscrew, Around the World targets your powerhouse (abs, inner thighs, and butt) while stretching your back and also improves balance and control. The twisting aspect of this exercise adds an extra element of control. Before attempting this exercise, make sure that you've mastered the regular Rollover (Chapter 7) and the Corkscrew (Chapter 7).

Around the World can put a lot of stress on your neck. Avoid this exercise if you have a neck injury.

Getting set

Lie on your back and place a small ball or magic circle between your ankles. Straighten your legs up to the sky and place your arms, palms down, by your sides, pressing your arms down on the mat. Allow your legs to drop so they make a 45-degree angle with the floor.

The exercise

Inhale: Pull your belly in and squeeze your butt to lift your legs up and over your head so that your legs are parallel to the floor behind you. Push your arms into the floor to help you get your hips up. Keep your shoulders down away from the ears. Don't roll back onto your neck. Instead, balance between your shoulder blades.

Exhale: Figure 12-6 shows the circular movement of the legs that you perform on the exhale that gives Around the World its name. To start the movement, twist your hips slightly to the right and let your legs begin to circle down to the left. Roll down the left side of your spine. Push your arms into the floor to facilitate this movement. As you roll down your spine, allow your legs to continue the circle, dropping them down and then up to the right and completing the circle with your legs as you roll up the right side of your spine.

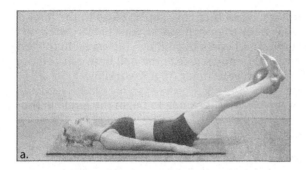

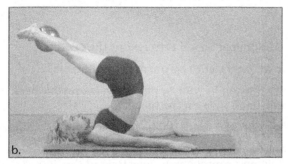

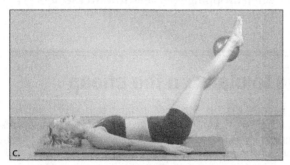

Figure 12-6:
Around the
World.

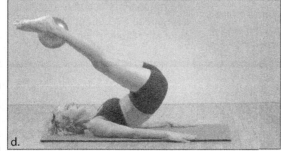

When circling your legs, allow them to drop as close to the floor as you can without allowing your belly to pooch out or your back to arch off the mat. Keep your torso stable at all costs by pulling your navel in toward your spine and squeezing your butt! Gently squeeze the ball between your legs during the whole exercise to keep your inner thighs working.

Inhale at the top of the circle and exhale to begin the circle in the opposite direction.

Complete 6 repetitions, alternating directions. Finish by bringing your knees into your chest.

Do's and don'ts

- ✔ Do keep your Abdominal Scoop throughout the exercise.

- ✔ Do use your arms for stability by pushing into the mat.

- ✔ Do minimize the tension in your upper body; keep your neck long and relaxed and your back wide on the mat.

- ✔ Do squeeze your butt and inner thighs together to help stabilize the core.

- ✔ Don't allow your back to arch off the mat at all! Keep your lower back flat on the mat when dropping your legs toward the floor. Try for absolute stability here.

Going to class on the cheap

There's a myth out there that Pilates classes cost you a well-toned arm and a leg. Not true! You can find classes — including classes that use the magic circle or a small ball — at reasonable rates.

One thing to remember is that you can find a Pilates mat class at just about every gym nowadays, and sometimes the cost is even included in your membership fee! If you're already a member, it's free Pilates instruction. Also, at fully equipped Pilates studios, you may be able to find group classes on the Pilates equipment or with Pilates accessories. Although extensive one-on-one instruction is admittedly outside of many people's budget, group classes can be quite affordable.

Chapter 13

Size Does Matter: Exercises on the Big Ball

- -

- -

*T*he fitness ball — basically a big, bouncy ball — was supposedly developed by a physical therapist in Europe who wanted injured patients to be able to get some aerobic conditioning. The therapist put patients on the ball and had them bounce. Eureka — the patients got a great workout without impacting their injuries.

Fitness balls are still used by physical therapists and Pilates teachers to rehabilitate back, knee, and hip injuries, but they can do a whole lot more. The big balls can really make exercise fun, and they can be a great tool to help you learn core stability, balance, control, and strength.

Sitting on a ball instead of a chair is a great way to keep your spine healthy. I recommend trying to sit on a ball for at least part of your work day, if you have a desk job. When you sit on a ball, you're forced to sit up with good posture because you have nothing to lean back on. Also, because the ball rolls around, it keeps you on your toes and keeps your body moving, which helps prevent the stiffness and back pain that you can get from being too sedentary.

The ball rolls around easily, so core strength and balance are required to keep it still — much like with the roller (see Chapter 11 for more on the roller). The challenge of keeping the ball still makes the ball an excellent tool to teach stability and rehabilitation. The simplest movement can become a huge challenge when you do it on the ball.

If you have a ball, you can incorporate the exercises mentioned in this chapter as an addition to your Pilates workout. Using a ball can give your workout a little more variety and extra challenge. You can try these exercises after your Pilates mat work.

Fitness balls come in different sizes. My basic rule for choosing the correct size is that when you're sitting on the ball, you should be able to easily balance with your feet on the ground. Your hips and knees should both be at right angles. The following list matches you up with the right size ball, based on your height:

- ✔ 55 centimeters if you're under 5 feet tall
- ✔ 65 centimeters if you're between 5 feet and 5 feet 7 inches tall
- ✔ 75 centimeters if you're between 5 feet 8 inches and 6 feet 2 inches tall
- ✔ 85 centimeters if you're over 6 feet 2 inches tall

A great place to buy fitness balls is The Gym Ball Store. You can contact the store on the Web at www.gymballstore.com or by phone at 1-800-393-7255.

After you buy your ball, blow it up so that it gives a little when it's pushed, but not so much that it feels soggy. My friend Carol actually blew up her fitness ball with her mouth, but I recommend a bicycle pump, a foot pump, or, for the fastest inflation, a gas station's tire pump.

Note: I include the level of difficulty next to the name of each exercise in this chapter.

Exercises in This Chapter

My studio offers ball classes that combine an aerobic workout with lots of tough abdominal and upper body exercises. The exercises in this chapter are some of the favorites in my studio:

- ✔ Roll Downs
- ✔ Upper Abdominal Curls
- ✔ Open Back Stretch
- ✔ Bridge on the Ball
- ✔ Plank on the Ball
- ✔ Knees to Chest
- ✔ The Up Stretch
- ✔ Lana Turner Stretch

Roll Downs (Beginning)

This exercise tests your stability and warms up your belly and your back. Make sure that you have bare feet or sneakers or some traction for your feet, or you may slip and fall off your ball. If you have slippery bare feet, you may want to moisten them if you're on a smooth surface, or try this exercise on a rug instead.

If you're a bit rusty on your Pilates alphabet, you may want to take a quick look at Chapter 3. C Curve, Bridge, Abdominal Scoop, and Stacking the Spine are all elements of the alphabet that appear in this exercise.

Getting set

Sit up tall on the ball with your feet a little wider than hip distance apart. Reach your arms straight out in front of you so that they're approximately parallel with your hips (Figure 13-1a).

The exercise

Exhale: Pull your navel in toward your spine and begin to roll down your spine, thinking of pulling the ball forward with your tailbone as you round your lower back into a C Curve. Slowly step your feet forward to accommodate the movement of your body (Figure 13-1b). Roll all the way down until your upper back and shoulders are on the ball, with your body making a Bridge position — your feet planted firmly on the floor, your butt squeezing, and your belly pulled in to keep your hips at the same height as your shoulders.

Inhale: Reach your arms overhead, keeping your whole torso stable, and circle the arms open and then forward (Figures 13-1c and 13-1d).

Exhale: Begin to walk your feet backward toward the ball as you roll back up, using your deep Abdominal Scoop to help you control the movement. Finish by Stacking the Spine and sitting tall in the starting position, your arms reaching forward throughout.

Complete 4 repetitions. The last time you roll down, hold the Bridge position, put your hands behind your head, and go right into Upper Abdominal Curls.

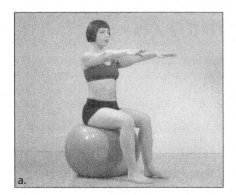
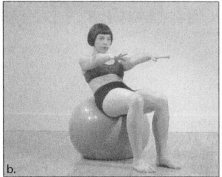
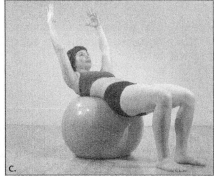
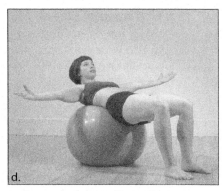

Figure 13-1:
Roll Downs.

Upper Abdominal Curls (Intermediate)

If you've already mastered Upper Abdominal Curls on the mat and want to *really* feel a burn in your belly, try them on the big ball. To stabilize on the ball, you must find your deep Abdominal Scoop! This is one of the most challenging abdominal exercises you'll find anywhere.

The farther your pelvis is from the ball, the easier the exercise. If you need to make this exercise easier, walk your feet away from the ball so that your shoulders are making contact with the ball. Do the curls from this position.

Getting set

If you hold your last Bridge from the Roll Downs, you're in the right position. You should be lying back with your mid back making contact with the ball, your feet planted firmly on the floor a little more than hip distance apart, knees facing slightly away from each other. Squeeze your butt and pull your belly in to keep your hips at the same height as your shoulders. Make your torso as stable as possible.

Now, interlace your fingers and put your hands behind your head.

The exercise

Exhale: Make sure that your butt is squeezed and your navel is pulled in. Roll up to your Pilates Abdominal Position (Figure 13-2). Raise your head just high enough that your shoulder blades are off the ball. Don't let your hips drop down as you roll your upper body up.

Don't bounce up and down, but go slowly to really get the benefits of this exercise.

Inhale: Control the movement back down to the Bridge position.

Complete 8 repetitions slowly, and go right into your Open Back Stretch. Believe me — after this exercise, you'll need it!

Do's and don'ts

- ✔ Do think of pulling your belly so far in that you flatten your lower back onto the ball as you initiate the roll up. You're not in Neutral Spine during this exercise.

- ✔ Don't strain your neck. Allow your hands to hold the weight of your head and keep the space of a tangerine between your chin and your neck.

Modifications

To make the exercise more difficult, walk your feet in and start with your pelvis and lower back making contact with the ball. Stabilizing is more difficult when your belly is actually on top of the ball as you roll up. Think of flattening your lower back onto the ball as you initiate the roll up (Figure 13-3).

You can also modify the exercise to work your oblique abdominals (the deep abdominals that twist your torso). Instead of rolling straight up, try rolling up with a slight twist, reaching your right elbow toward your left knee and then reaching your left elbow toward your right knee, alternating sides every time.

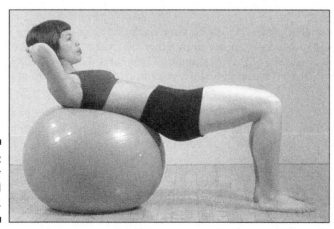

Figure 13-2:
Upper
Abdominal
Curls.

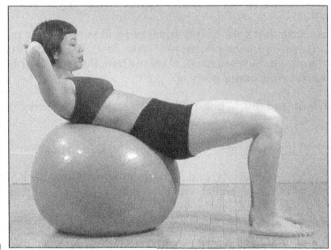

Figure 13-3:
Modifying Upper Abdominal Curls by moving the feet in.

Move your feet in to make the exercise more difficult.

Open Back Stretch (Intermediate)

This is a wonderful stretch for your chest muscles (your pectorals), shoulders, belly, and arms, and it's a great release for your back. People usually sigh or moan when they do this stretch because it feels so good. It's exactly what your spine needs after a day of working at a computer, nursing a baby, carrying heavy objects, or just living on earth with its silly gravitational forces. Open Back Stretch is sure to become one of your favorites!

Coming in and out of this exercise requires a fair amount of center strength and balance. Make sure that you can do Roll Downs on the fitness ball before attempting this exercise.

Getting set

Start from the Bridge position, with your back on the ball and your feet on the ground. You can get there from rolling down, as in the Roll Downs on the fitness ball. If you just did the Upper Abdominal Curls on the fitness ball, you're ready to go. Make sure that when you start, your upper back is on top of the ball.

The exercise

Inhale: Keeping your feet planted on the floor a little wider than hip distance apart, push back with your legs, reaching your arms above your head and toward the floor behind you.

Keep your feet in contact with the floor, or you might roll off the ball!

Breathing continuously: Slowly circle your arms, allowing the weight of your arms to hang heavy toward the floor to really open up the chest (Figure 13-4a). Let your arms open to the sides, down by your body. Cross your arms as if you're taking off a sweater and then reach them again above your head.

If you find a spot while you're circling your arms that feels in particular need of a stretch, hold this position and take a deep breath.

Think of expanding the chest on the inhale to increase the stretch.

Complete 2 repetitions reverse the circle for 2 repetitions.

To finish, slowly roll forward, your arms down by your sides, until you're squatting (Figure 13-4b). Allow your knees and feet to turn out and adjust underneath you so that you can come to a deep knee bend while keeping both feet entirely on the floor. You may need to widen your stance to keep your heels down.

Keep your back glued to the fitness ball so that your head is still released back, your chest is open, and the weight of your head and neck is supported by the ball. Hold the squat for 10 seconds as you allow the blood to flow out of your head. If you come up too fast, you may get dizzy.

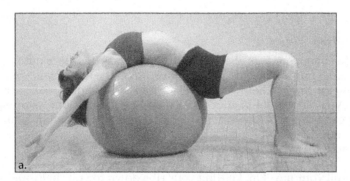

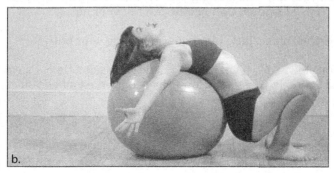

Figure 13-4:
Open Back
Stretch.

Slowly lift your head (you can put your hands behind your head to lift it) and begin to roll back up your spine, walking your feet toward the ball, reaching your arms forward, and using your abdominals to control the movement back up. End by sitting up tall on your ball.

Bridge on the Ball (Beginning)

I describe how to do the Bridge in the beginning mat series (Chapter 5) and with the small ball (Chapter 12). Here's a variation with the big ball. Like the other Bridges, this exercise is an excellent exercise to strengthen your butt and the back of your legs, and it teaches core stability. Doing the Bridge on the big ball adds an extra element of stability, because stopping the ball from rolling around takes a lot of control.

Getting set

Lie on your back with your arms by your sides and your legs straight and resting up on the ball (Figure 13-5a). The closer the ball is to your body, the easier it is to stabilize, so start with the ball close to you. Your calves and knees should be resting on the ball the first time you try this exercise. As you get stronger, you can start with the ball farther away from you. Inhale deeply to begin.

The exercise

Exhale: Keeping your legs absolutely straight, press your legs onto the ball and squeeze your butt as you lift your hips up off the mat. Press your arms and palms into the floor to help you stabilize. Your body should make a straight line from your shoulders to your toes (Figure 13-5b). Don't press up so high that you can't see your knees or so high that you bear weight on your neck.

Inhale: Hold this Bridge position.

Exhale: Pull your navel in, knitting your ribs down to your belly and squeezing your butt. Try to lengthen through the front of your hips.

Inhale: Lift your hips a little higher by squeezing your butt.

Exhale: Roll slowly down your spine one vertebra at a time. Use the Abdominal Scoop to press your lower back onto the mat as you come back to Neutral Spine.

Complete 5 repetitions.

Transition by bringing your knees into your chest to relax your back.

Modification

Do the one-legged Bridge shown in Figures 13-6a and 13-6b. Come up to the Bridge position, lift one leg up to the sky, allowing your knee to bend, and then straighten it. Hold for 1 breath and then place the leg back on the ball, reaching it long as it returns to the ball. Square your hips and switch sides.

Do's and don'ts

- ✔ Do maintain a straight position when you're up in the Bridge. Try not to arch your back.

- ✔ Do attempt to articulate through your spine on the way down.

- ✔ Do minimize the tension in your upper body; keep your neck long and relaxed.

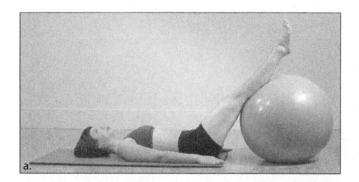

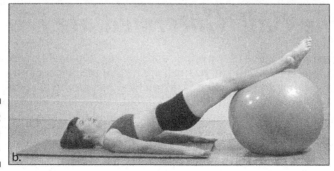

Figure 13-5:
Bridge on
the Ball.

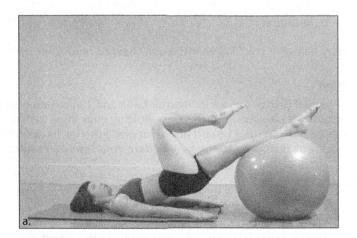

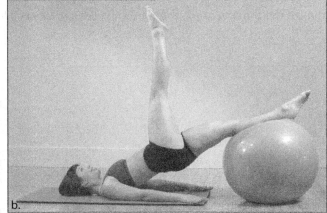

Figure 13-6:
The one-legged variation of Bridge on the Ball.

Plank on the Ball (Intermediate)

Now you're starting some of the upper body strengthening. Many of these upper body exercises on the fitness ball are a great preparation for gymnastics and yoga. If you regularly practice Plank on the Ball and the next two exercises, Knees to Chest and The Up Stretch, you'll build a great amount of upper body strength. Plank on the Ball is similar to the advanced mat exercise Control Front (see Chapter 7). Make sure that you've mastered Control Front on the mat before attempting this exercise.

Getting set

Lie with your belly on the ball and your palms planted down on the floor (Figure 13-7a). Keep your arms shoulder distance apart and your fingers facing forward. Lift your legs up in line with your torso so that your whole body makes a rigid plank, squeezing your legs together from the inner thighs, pulling your navel in, and squeezing your butt to keep the center supported.

Walk your hands away from the ball, but only as far as you can while still controlling the plank position from your belly and butt. The farther you walk away from the ball, the more center strength is required to maintain the position. Don't let your lower back sag down, but tuck your pelvis under and pull your belly up to support your lower back. Ultimately, you want to walk your hands out to the point where your knees are on top of the ball, as shown in Figure 13-7b.

You're a wooden plank, and someone is stepping up onto the middle of your back. Press up from your arms, pull up from your belly, and squeeze your butt to resist this imaginary weight.

The exercise

Breathing continuously: Maintain your rigid plank position and keep your arms straight, your palms planted on the floor, and your fingers spread. Rock forward and back a few inches in each direction, all the while maintaining your rigid plank (Figure 13-7c).

Complete 8 repetitions of this rocking motion and then walk your hands back toward the ball and lie forward, letting your head release forward into a nice relaxed stretch on the ball.

Modification

Once you're out in your plank position, do 8 push-ups. Exhale on the way down and inhale on the way up. Count to three in each direction so that you aren't just popping up and down. Keep your neck long.

Adjust the placement of your body on the ball to accommodate your strength level. The closer your torso is to the ball, the easier the exercise. As you develop core strength, try walking all the way out to your feet!

Do's and don'ts

- ✔ Do keep the top of your head reaching long in front of you.

- ✔ Do keep squeezing your butt and pulling your navel in, using your Abdominal Scoop throughout the exercise.

- ✔ Don't let your shoulders hunch up by your ears, but keep your shoulder blades pulling down your back.

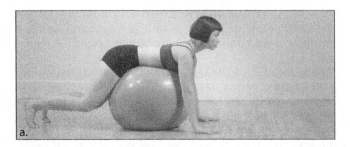

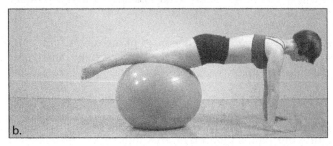

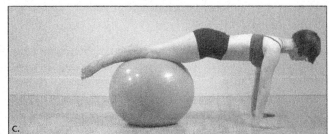

Figure 13-7:
Plank on
the Ball.

Rock a few inches forward and back.

Knees to Chest (Intermediate)

This exercise combines an upper body workout with abdominal work and a
back stretch. It feels good, and it's fun to do!

Getting set

The setup is the same as the Plank on the Ball. Start by lying with your belly
on the ball and your palms planted down on the floor (Figure 13-8a). Keep
your arms shoulder distance apart and your fingers facing forward. Lift your

legs up in line with your torso so that your whole body makes a rigid plank, squeezing your legs together from your inner thighs, pulling your navel in, and squeezing your butt to keep the center supported.

Walk your hands away from the ball, maintaining your plank position, so that your knees are on top of the ball (Figure 13-8b).

Make sure that you start in the proper position for this exercise. The knees must be on top of the center of the ball. If you're too close to the ball, you won't have enough space to do the movement. If you're too far from the ball, you'll probably roll off the ball onto the floor!

The exercise

Inhale: Lift your hips up by scooping your belly in, and pull your knees into your chest, making a fetus shape on top of the ball. Think of pulling the ball forward with your knees as your hips rise up. Keep your arms straight and strong. Figures 13-8c and 13-8d show this movement.

Exhale: Come back to the plank position.

Complete 8 repetitions. Then walk your arms back to the ball and rest by lying forward over the ball.

Modification

You can work your obliques by doing the same exercise as Knees to Chest, except instead of pulling your knees straight into your chest, send your knees slightly off center as they come in toward your body, making a circular motion with the ball. Then come into your fetal position on top of the ball and, on the way back, complete your circular shape by sending your knees in the opposite direction. Figures 13-9a and 13-9b show the circular movement.

If the ball had paint on it, it would paint one large oval shape on the floor from beginning to end.

Make sure that you really lift your hips and scoop your belly up and in to initiate the movement of the knees, or you may find yourself falling off the ball.

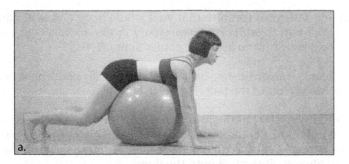

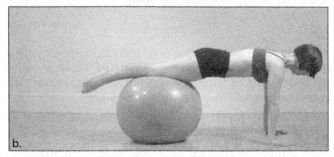

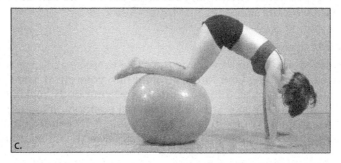

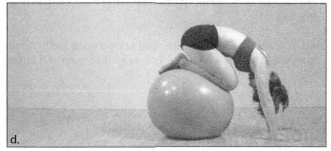

Figure 13-8:
Knees to
Chest.

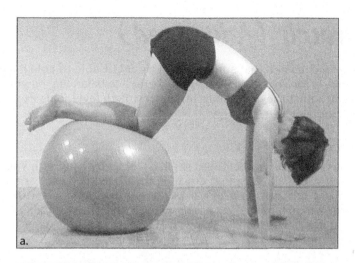

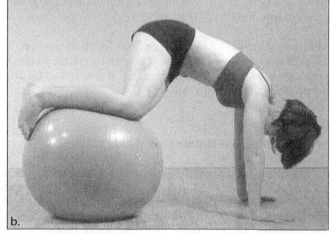

Figure 13-9:
Modifying
Knees to
Chest to
work the
obliques.

The Up Stretch (Advanced)

If you've ever dreamed that someday you would be able to hold a handstand, this exercise is for you. It's a great way to practice balancing on your arms, and you can adjust the position to fit your strength level. This exercise builds deep belly and back strength and teaches balance on the arms.

Getting set

The setup is the same as the Knees to Chest. Start by lying with your belly on the ball with your palms planted down on the floor. Keep your arms shoulder distance apart, fingers facing forward. Lift your legs up in line with your torso so that your whole body makes a rigid plank, squeezing your legs together from your inner thighs, pulling your navel in, and squeezing your butt to keep the center supported.

Walk your hands away from the ball, maintaining your plank position, so that your knees are on top of the ball (Figure 13-10a).

Make sure that you start in the proper position for this exercise. The knees must be on top of the center of the ball. If you're too close to the ball, you won't have enough space to do the movement. If you're too far from the ball, you may end up doing a front flip onto the floor!

The exercise

Inhale: Breathe deeply and maintain your plank.

Exhale: Lift your hips up by scooping your belly in and fold your body in half (Figure 13-10b). Think of pulling the ball forward with your knees as your hips rise up. Keep your arms and legs straight and strong and think of pushing away from the floor with your arms. Think of a Jackknife movement, where the body folds in the middle in one percussive movement, making an inverted V shape.

Inhale: Come back to the plank position.

Repeat 8 times. Then walk your arms back to the ball and rest by lying forward over the ball.

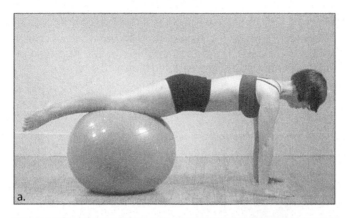

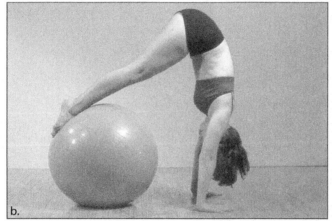

Figure 13-10:
The Up
Stretch.

Lana Turner Stretch (Beginning)

This exercise was named by a client of mine who saw the resemblance to the popular bathing beauty of years past. Lana Turner is a great stretch for the sides of your body.

Getting set

Start in the mermaid position, sitting on the side of your hip, with your knees bent, legs folded on top of each other, and your top foot in front. Put one hand on the side of your head and lean the side of your ribs and your armpit against the ball with your elbow up, as shown in Figure 13-11a, finding a place to balance. Relax your other hand in front of you or on your legs.

If you don't feel a stretch in the side of your body, try moving a little away from the ball so that your ribs can really drop down as your arm stays propped up on the ball.

The stretch

Breathe and hold the stretch for 30 seconds. To vary the stretch, slowly roll your ribs back and forward, holding the positions and finding a new stretch in each position, as shown in Figures 13-11b and 13-11c.

Repeat the exercise on the other side.

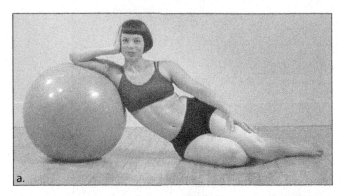

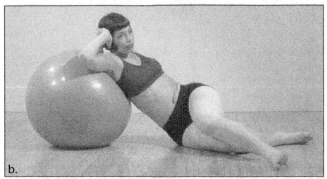

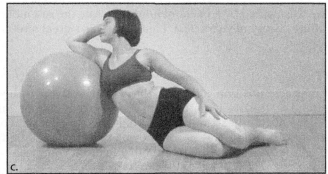

Figure 13-11:
Lana Turner
Stretch.

Chapter 14

Hitting the Wall for a Pilates Cool-Down

Many people have lost the ability to stand up straight with their head in proper alignment, balanced on top of their hips. These people have what I call forward-head posture. If you feel a strange stretch or pull when you stand with your back and head against a wall, then you probably have forward-head posture. This posture is a natural effect of sitting at a computer for hours at a time, or of just generally slumping while sitting and standing in daily life.

Pilates wall exercises help to reverse this forward-head phenomena and are classically considered a cool-down in the Pilates method. These exercises can also be done on their own as a set for anyone needing a gentle reminder of what proper posture should feel like.

I was originally taught to do these exercises with a 1- or 2-pound free weight in each hand. If you don't own weights, don't worry; you can do these exercises without any accessory at all. All you need is an open wall with enough space to spread your arms up and open.

Wall Exercises in This Chapter

There aren't many wall exercises in this chapter — just the best ones I know:

✔ Arm Circles on the Wall

✔ Squats Against the Wall

✔ Rolling Down the Wall

Arm Circles on the Wall

Arm Circles on the Wall is a great way to align and stretch out your shoulders. This may seem like a wimpy exercise — "Hey, I'm just moving my arms around." But the point of this exercise is *proprioception,* which means how the brain perceives where you are in space. In this case, focus on the feeling of having your spine straight with your head in its proper upright position. The motion of your arms gives valuable information to your brain as to where your upper body should be in space. Believe me, it's not as easy as it looks!

Getting set

Stand with your back against the wall, your knees soft, and your feet hip distance apart. Try to maintain Neutral Spine by pressing your tailbone into the wall and by keeping a small space between your lower back and the wall. Your arms should be hanging down by your sides. If you have 1- or 2-pound dumbbells, hold one in each hand.

When I say make your knees soft, that just means bend them slightly. I prefer "soft" because it gives you a better idea of what you're aiming for.

Take a deep breath.

The exercise

Exhale: Feel your shoulders dropping down away from your ears as you slowly lift your arms straight forward, pressing your shoulder blades against the wall (Figure 14-1a).

Inhale: Keep lifting your arms until they're all the way up by your ears, allowing your arms to touch the wall above you. Try not to let your upper back arch off the wall (Figure 14-1b).

Exhale: Keeping your arms on the wall, make a circle with them. Imagine that you're cleaning the walls with your arms. Finish the circle with the arms back by your sides (Figure 14-1c).

Complete 2 repetitions and reverse. Reverse the circle by moving your arms up from your side as if you're making angels in the snow. When your arms reach up by your ears, bring your arms forward, keeping them shoulder distance apart, and think of pressing your shoulder blades back against the wall. Finish with your arms back by your sides.

Do's and don'ts

- ✔ Do keep your whole spine against the wall.
- ✔ Don't let your shoulders rise up by your ears, but keep them dropping down your back.

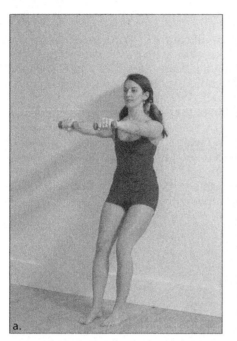

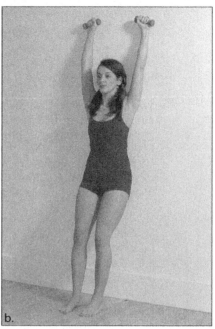

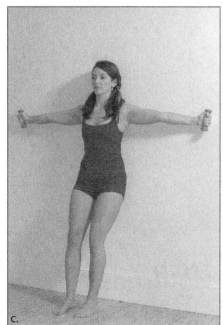

Figure 14-1:
Arm Circles
on the Wall.

Modification

Chicken Wings is a fabulous modification of Arm Circles on the Wall. The simple addition of bending your elbows on the way down helps to further open up your chest, stretching out those pectorals while engaging the muscles that are necessary to hold the shoulders in their proper alignment.

Start by reversing the direction of the Arm Circles. Lift your arms open to the sides first, then drag them up by your ears. When your arms are reaching straight up, bend your elbows, trying to keep your arms in contact with the wall. Slowly allow your elbows to lead the way down, making a right angle with your arm, as shown in Figure 14-2. When you can't pull your elbows down any farther, allow your arms to straighten and come back down by your sides, and then start over. Complete 3 repetitions.

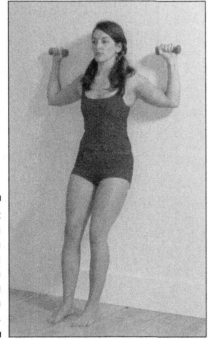

Figure 14-2:
Doing the
Chicken
Wing
modification
of Arm
Circles on
the Wall.

Squats Against the Wall

Squats Against the Wall work your legs and butt while helping to align your spine and improve posture.

Getting set

Stand with your back against the wall and your feet 2 "feet" away from the wall — measure two of *your* feet and set up that distance from the wall, rather than 24 inches from the wall. Keep your feet hip distance apart. Try to maintain Neutral Spine by pressing your tailbone into the wall while keeping a small space between your lower back and the wall. Your arms should be hanging down by your sides. If you have 1- or 2-pound dumbbells, hold one in each hand, your arms hanging down by your sides.

The exercise

Breathing slowly and continuously: Begin the squat by sliding down the wall, keeping Neutral Spine. Keep your legs parallel with each other by making sure that your knees don't roll in or out but stay aligned with the middle toes.

Slide down to where you feel some work in your legs and butt, but no farther than you would be able to if you had a chair beneath you. You may need to adjust your legs farther away from the wall to go down into the full squat. Think of pressing into your heels to help activate the muscles in the back of your legs and butt.

Bring your arms up straight in front of you and hold them there, and hold the squat for 3 full breaths. Your position should be similar to that of the model in Figure 14-3. You can increase the length of the squat as you get stronger. Slide back up the wall and rest for 1 breath. Complete 3 to 5 repetitions.

Never bend your knees past 90 degrees when you perform a squat. Doing so puts too much pressure on your knee joints.

Do's and don'ts

- ✔ Do keep your whole spine against the wall.
- ✔ Do keep pressing your heels into the floor to cue the back of your legs and butt.

Modifications

You can add the element of moving your arms. After you're in the squat position, with your arms straight ahead, you can bend your elbows in toward the wall while keeping your forearms forward. You should look like a boxer pulling back for a punch. Then extend your arms back to the starting position, straight out in front of you, as if you're punching someone in front of you with both fists. Figure 14-4 shows this modification.

For another variation, change the position of your legs. Try the same squat with your legs open wide and turned out and your knees facing away from each other. As you slide down the wall, you still want to keep your knees aligned over your middle toes. This means you must keep working the turn-out from the hips.

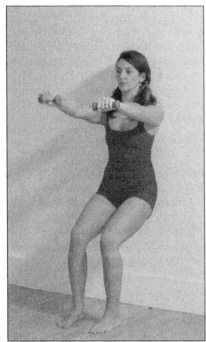

Figure 14-3:
Squats
Against the
Wall.

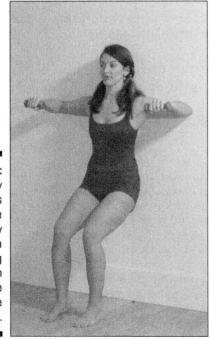

Figure 14-4:
Modify
Squats
Against the
Wall by
making a
punching
motion
while
holding the
squat.

Rolling Down the Wall

Rolling Down the Wall is a nice way to finish your workout because it teaches the body where vertical is, and you can walk away from the exercise feeling like your posture is perfect. Rolling Down the Wall stretches out your whole back: the neck, upper back, and lower back.

Getting set

Stand with your back against the wall, your knees soft, and your feet hip distance apart and facing forward, about 6 inches to a foot away from the wall. Try to maintain Neutral Spine by pressing your tailbone into the wall while keeping a small space between your lower back and the wall. Your arms should be hanging down by your sides. If you have 1- or 2-pound dumbbells, hold one in each hand (Figure 14-5a).

The exercise

Breathing slowly and continuously: Begin rolling down the wall by letting your head slowly drop forward, feeling the stretch in the back of your neck. Then peel your spine off the wall one vertebra at a time, allowing your arms to drop forward with the weight of the dumbbells (or just the weight of your arms). Figures 14-5b and 14-5c show the model dropping forward. Don't worry if you're not quite as limber as she is!

Once you've dropped as far forward as you feel able to drop with your hips still against the wall, make gentle circles with your arms as they hang heavy with gravity. Allow the circles to come to a stop, and begin to roll back up the wall, lifting from your belly and adjusting the bend in your knees so that you can press the lower back into the wall as you begin your roll up. Try to press each vertebra into the wall as you slowly Stack the Spine. Your arms will hang forward as you roll up. Keep your head hanging heavy until the very end. Finish the exercise by standing in the starting position, in Neutral Spine, your arms by your sides.

You're now officially cooled down and ready to stand up and go about your business feeling taller and more aligned.

Do's and don'ts

> ✔ Do keep your belly scooped in to support the stretch of your back.

> ✔ Do keep your knees soft and your hips always against the wall.

> ✔ Do keep breathing slowly as you gradually get your stretch.

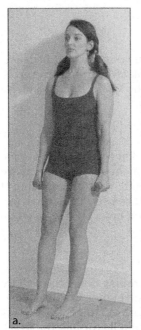 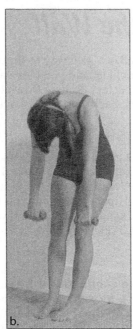

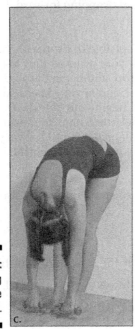

Figure 14-5:
Rolling
Down the
Wall.

Chapter 15

Springs Are Busting Out All Over: An Overview of Pilates Equipment

"Wow, that looks scary."

"Does that hurt?"

"Hey, that looks like the rack!"

*W*hen people first set their eyes on Pilates equipment, these are the kinds of things they invariably say. And I have to counter with a smile and assure them that Pilates equipment is some of the most comfortable and relaxing equipment in existence.

In this chapter, I give you an overview of Pilates equipment just to familiarize you with what's out there. You may be seduced enough by the Pilates mat work to want to go to your local Pilates studio and hop on a reformer so that you can explore even more of what Pilates has to offer. I don't go into details about specific exercises, because that would be a whole other book. I'm assuming that you don't have any equipment at the moment, so this book focuses on the mat work and simple accessories that are inexpensive to buy.

Buying a large piece of Pilates equipment is an investment in both money and space. But it can be worth it. If you're curious about trying the equipment after reading this chapter, check out your local Pilates studio. I don't recommend buying anything until you've had the chance to try it more than just a few times first.

If you do decide to buy a piece of equipment, don't attempt to use it without the guidance of a certified instructor or a good video. I recommend getting some personal instruction first and using a video later to assist you with your home workout once you understand the basics. Learning the correct form is essential, especially when on the equipment, because you can easily injure yourself.

For all your Pilates needs, including a list of Pilates instructors and studios in your area and a catalog of good videos, accessories, and equipment, call Balanced Body at 1-800-745-2837 (1-800-PILATES). Press 0 then extension 10. Balanced Body manufactures excellent equipment, which is featured in my studios and in the photos in this chapter. You can also visit the company on the Web at www.pilates.com.

Why Equipment?

If you've been doing the Pilates mat work diligently, you may wonder why anyone needs special equipment. After all, the mat is enough of a workout! Well, the equipment adds a whole other dimension to Pilates work, and can be quite fun to boot.

For help with basic movements

The story goes that Joe Pilates invented his equipment to replace himself as a spotter for his clients. Joe got tired of pulling people up who were unable to do a sit-up by themselves. So he invented the roll-back bar. The roll-back bar (from the Pilates Spring Board or cadillac) consists of a wooden dowel that has two fairly strong springs attached to it. The dowel, in turn, is fastened to a wall or structure against which you can easily roll up and down. Suppose that you can't do a Roll Up (an exercise from Chapter 6) by yourself. The roll-back bar can assist you with it and make it possible to complete a movement that would otherwise be impossible. Not only can you now complete this previously unattainable Roll Up, but the assistance of the springs allows you to complete the movement smoothly, with articulation and control.

The springs act as abdominal muscles that you do not yet have. As you get stronger and stronger, the spring resistance can be diminished so that your abdominal muscles can slowly do more and more of the work, until — voilà — you're able to do a full Roll Up all by yourself!

For help doing the exotic stuff

The equipment can enable you to experience all kinds of wacky positions that otherwise only an acrobat could perform. If you don't believe me, look at the photos in this chapter.

For strengthening the limbs

The mat work focuses mainly on core strength: abs, butt, and back. The equipment, however, combines core training with strength training for your legs, hips, arms, shoulders, and inner thighs. The machines give you full-body resistance training, much like a weightlifting routine, but don't bulk you up — as I explain in the next section.

For long, lean muscles

If you're lucky enough to work out on the Pilates equipment, you'll notice your muscles gaining strength and tone without increasing in bulk. This result is due to the springs that are used in Pilates equipment. A spring's resistance increases along a continuum — as a spring stretches, it becomes more and more taut. The muscle that is challenging the spring is challenged along this continuum.

When you first pull on a spring, it may have 5 pounds of resistance, but by the time you've stretched it all the way out, it may have 10 pounds of resistance. The muscle that is working to pull that spring will be affected by this change. Working the muscles along a continuum builds long, strong, and supple muscles, whereas working out with free weights or doing impact sports creates a bigger, bulkier, tighter muscle. The sidebar "Choosing between Pilates and weight training" has more information.

For emphasizing control

After you stretch out a spring, it wants to shorten back to its original resting length. When doing a Pilates exercise against this resistance, you must work to bring the spring back home to its original length slowly and carefully — *with control.* When working on Pilates equipment, you must always control the movement on the return portion of an exercise. If you're straightening your legs out against resistance, for example, you must control the movement back to the starting position, with your legs bent. When you train your body to control the movement that extends the spring and that contracts it, you train your body to have greater balance and control in general.

Choosing between Pilates and weight training

I recently spoke another Pilates professional who just got back from a fitness conference. He told me that he saw many former weight lifters walking around and that they looked terrible. Their muscles had deflated and turned to flab, and many were overweight. This is the trouble with weight lifting: You build up bulk in your muscles that must be maintained by constant training. The moment you stop lifting weights, the muscles lose their tone. The skin has expanded to hold the bigger mass. As the muscles shrink, the skin sags.

Not so in Pilates. As you build muscle tone with spring resistance, your muscles will not bulk up but will probably become longer and more toned without increasing very much in size (depending on the size of the muscle when you start). You will notice definition without bulk. Your muscles will learn to work more efficiently, and your movements will become more graceful. You don't have to constantly train to keep the tone (although, of course, you will lose some tone if you completely stop training for a long time).

But the main difference between Pilates and weight training is that Pilates exercises are complete movements that require many muscles to work at once, while weight training works muscles in isolation.

Even if you're a high-level athlete, your day-to-day movements utilize many muscles at once. In Pilates, as in normal daily movements like climbing stairs or kneeling to pick up a child, you don't isolate one muscle but are always working many muscles together (called *synergy*). Therefore, one muscle will never become overdeveloped.

When I think of weight lifting, I think of one big muscle that has been worked in isolation and is just sitting there on your body, a big mass that you don't have any use for. You have to carry around this extra mass, even though it's not really helping you to function in your daily life. Carrying around that mass is an inefficient use of your body's resources.

Controlling both directions of a movement challenges the muscles while they're shortening (when you make the initial push against the spring, called *concentric contraction* of a muscle) and while they're lengthening (on the control portion of the movement, called *eccentric contraction* of a muscle). Eccentric training builds long and lean musculature.

A Rundown of the Equipment

Today, four main pieces of equipment are used in most studios:

- ✔ The universal reformer — probably the piece of equipment most often bought for individual use
- ✔ The wunda chair

> ✔ The cadillac (sometimes also called the trap table)
>
> ✔ The high barrel

I write about the reformer, wunda chair, and cadillac in more detail in the following sections. The high barrel is mainly used to stretch the legs and hips and is one of the least important pieces of Pilates equipment, so I don't go into any more detail about it. But I do write about a newly developed piece of equipment, called the Pilates Spring Board.

A medieval torture device with comfy upholstery: The universal reformer

The universal reformer, usually just called the reformer, is one of the most versatile pieces of Pilates equipment. When I first started my studio, all I had was one reformer and a mat. I was pretty happy with this setup for a few years, and I think my clients were happy, too. In fact, when I was first learning about Pilates while doing rehabilitation on my knee, I mainly did exercises on the reformer.

The reformer consists of a large wooden frame with tracks on either side on which sits a carriage that you can lie on or sit on. The carriage moves back and forth on the tracks. Attached to the carriage are five springs that you can modify based on the exercise. Attached to the frame is a foot bar that you press against to do leg-strengthening exercises. This foot bar makes the reformer the main piece of equipment for lower body strengthening and makes it an excellent device for knee, ankle, and hip rehabilitation. Straps are attached to the carriage that you can place on your feet or hands to create resistance training for your lower and upper body.

You can do hundreds of exercises on the reformer, and if I had to choose only one piece of equipment to own, I would definitely choose the reformer. The only drawback to the reformer is the price. Buying a studio-quality reformer will set you back about $2,500 to $3,000. You're paying for a hand-constructed apparatus of wood and metal springs that also includes high-quality ropes, neoprene handles, and cotton foot straps. These reformers are incredibly sturdy and come with a ten-year guarantee. I have owned one for almost ten years. Even though it's been used by clients daily throughout that period of time, it's had only minor maintenance. Old Bessie still works pretty darn good for all the wear and tear she's had!

In Figure 15-1, the model (yours truly) is demonstrating Control Front, an advanced exercise. The mat version of Control Front is in Chapter 7. This exercise strengthens your core, your upper body, your legs, and your butt. The carriage moves slightly back and forth in this exercise, and I control that movement from my abdominal muscles.

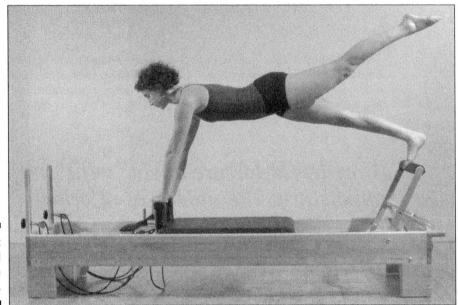

Figure 15-1:
Control
Front on the
reformer.

In Figure 15-2, I'm demonstrating Front Splits, another advanced exercise. This exercise increases flexibility in your legs and hips while toning and strengthening the front and back of your legs. This one is great for gymnasts in training.

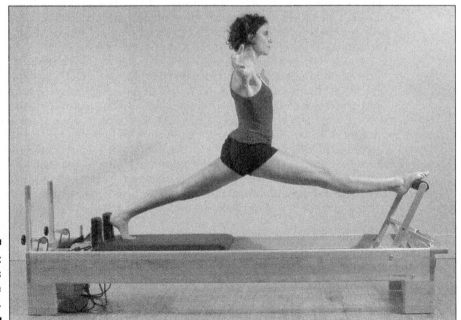

Figure 15-2:
Front Splits
on the
reformer.

It can double as a piece of furniture: The wunda chair

The wunda chair (German for *wonder chair; wunda* is pronounced *vunda*) looks unassuming enough — like an upholstered stool with a movable bar to one side of it — but it's one of the most difficult pieces of equipment to use. Even beginning exercises are fairly challenging on the wunda chair. In part, this is because the springs are extra heavy. Most of the exercises that have been developed for the wunda chair require a great amount of center strength and/or upper and lower body strength.

The wunda chair is great for gymnasts who are preparing for competition, or for those who want to develop the muscles of their back and shoulders. Because the wunda chair is oriented vertically, meaning that you sit or stand, as opposed to horizontally like the reformer and cadillac, it allows for a different kind of conditioning. Because you can re-create positions that are more common in daily life (sitting and standing), the exercises can be used for rehabilitation. The wunda chair adds some nice variety to your Pilates regimen. If you want one of your own, you can expect to pay $600 to $1,000. Figures 15-3 and 15-4 show the wunda chair in action.

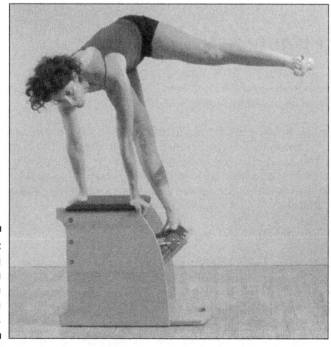

Figure 15-3: Side Leg Extension on the wunda chair.

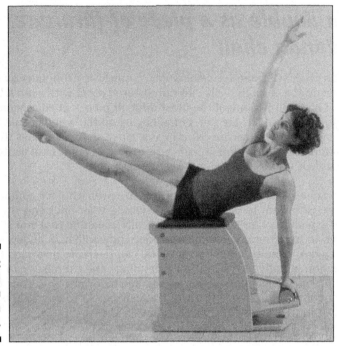

Figure 15-4:
Twisted
Teaser on
the wunda
chair.

Drivers wanted: The cadillac

The story goes that Joe Pilates mounted springs above hospital beds when he was a nurse in the army during World War II, and that the resulting apparatus was the mother of today's cadillac.

The cadillac has a trapeze that hangs from the top of the frame as a removable accessory. The trapeze gave the cadillac its original name, the trap table. Supposedly, the name changed one day when a little boy walked into the original Pilates studio in New York, looked at the trap table, and said, "Wow, that looks like a Cadillac!" The name stuck. Yes, this behemoth of a machine is a bit ostentatious.

Here are the features that you can find on a cadillac:

✔ **A wide bedlike base:** The bed is higher off the ground than the reformer, so injured and older people can get on and off easier. Because the bed is fairly large, the exercises are generally more comfortable for overweight and very tall people, and for people with tight muscles who can't put their bodies into small spaces.

✔ **Springs:** One end of the cadillac has various springs attached to it: two arm springs, two leg springs, and a roll-back bar.

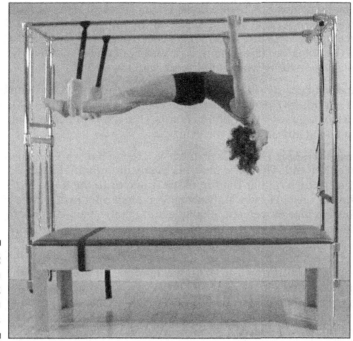

Figure 15-5:
Doing the
Open Back
Stretch on
the cadillac.

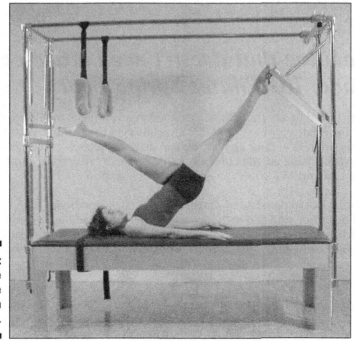

Figure 15-6:
Doing the
Reverse
Tower on
the cadillac.

✔ **A metal frame:** The bedlike base is framed on all sides with metal poles on each corner that are connected at the top, forming a three-dimensional rectangular structure 8 feet long, 2 feet wide, and 7 feet tall. You can climb on the poles and flip around, do a variety of pull-ups, or just hold on to the poles for security while doing work with the springs.

✔ **Fuzzies:** Fuzzies are tied to the top of the cadillac frame. These comfy little loops are for your feet while you hang upside down or hang horizontally with your hands holding the top of the frame. In Figure 15-5, I'm taking advantage of these fuzzies.

✔ **Push-thru bar:** The push-thru bar is a metal bar with two metal supports on either end. The bar can swing in any direction. The bar is supported by a spring to either the top of the frame or to the bottom of the frame. The bar has a circular path when you push on it from either direction. This circular movement is unique and creates very different exercises that can't be done on other pieces of equipment.

In Figure 15-6, I'm demonstrating the Reverse Tower, using the push-thru bar with a spring supporting it from above. In order for me to keep the bar in that position, I'm using a lot of core and butt strength. This is a slightly unusual exercise for the cadillac, as cadillac exercises are mostly geared for the upper body (shoulders, arms, abdominals, and back) with only a few exercises that focus on the legs and butt.

The cadillac, as you can imagine, will set you back a pretty penny — about $2,800 to $3,300.

A cadillac that doesn't need a two-car garage: The Pilates Spring Board

I'm very proud to say that I have designed my own piece of Pilates equipment! I call it the Pilates Spring Board. It's a variation of the cadillac that doesn't take up 16 square feet of floor space. You can do many exercises with it that you can do with a cadillac, plus lots more that you can't do on the cadillac. Figures 15-7 and 15-8 show the Spring Board in action.

The Spring Board consists of a large rectangular wood board with eyelets placed on either side at 6-inch increments. Like the cadillac, it comes with two arm springs, two leg springs, and a roll-back bar. But unlike the cadillac, you can adjust the height of the springs, from level with the floor to above your head, allowing for more exercise possibilities. You can do exercises lying on the mat, sitting up, kneeling, lunging, or standing. Many mat exercises can be modified so that the Pilates Spring Board adds to the challenge or facilitates the exercise. With the Pilates Spring Board, you can get full-body resistance training that strengthens your core, arms, legs, shoulders, butt, and back muscles.

Because the springs on the Spring Board are fairly heavy, your extremities get a fair amount of conditioning while your core is working overtime to stabilize against the rebound of a taut spring. You have to try it to know what I mean.

The Spring Board must be bolted into a wall — preferably into a stud — for support. This makes it perfect for an extra room, a home gym, garage, attic, or basement. It will cost you about $400. For more information, go to www.ellie.net. You can also ask me any general questions about equipment at my Web site.

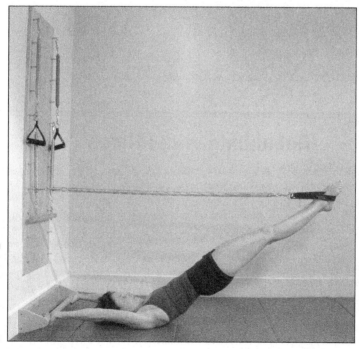

Figure 15-7:
Levitation
on the
Spring
Board.

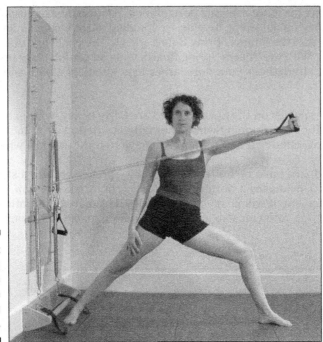

Figure 15-8:
Lunging
Swackadee
on the
Spring
Board.

Rehabbing with Pilates

When you're healing from an injury and are trying to regain strength in a weakened or destabilized area, beginning strength training very carefully is key. Pilates equipment is perfectly designed for this situation because it uses springs for resistance.

A spring increases its resistance along a continuum just as a joint increases its strength along a continuum. In other words, it's not great to put a big load on a joint when it's fully bent. You've probably experienced this concept when you try to stand up from a deep squat. You know how that movement can hurt your knees? It's because your knees aren't their most stable when you're in a deep squat.

When you initiate a movement against a slack spring, your joint or muscle is barely challenged, making the movement safe for an injured knee joint. As you straighten out your leg, the spring becomes increasingly more stretched out, increasing its resistance as it becomes more and more taut. But because your knee joint becomes less vulnerable as the leg straightens, the increased resistance is a safe and a welcome challenge.

Another advantage of Pilates equipment is that it allows the body to regain functional movement capability after injury. Functional movements are movements that replicate daily life activities such as walking, sitting, getting up, bending over, twisting around, and lying down.

Part IV
Special Situations

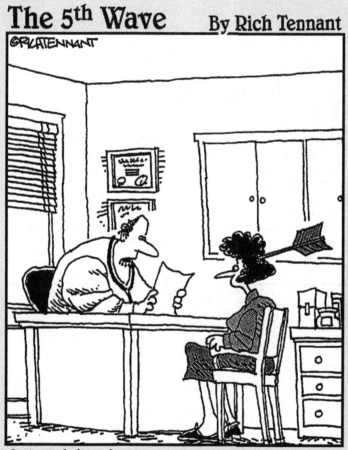

The 5th Wave   By Rich Tennant

"Well, Pilates is good for your health, but we may want to take a different approach to curing your constant headaches."

In this part . . .

You may need a special Pilates routine. If you're pregnant or were pregnant recently, check out Chapter 16. Even though you can't do all the exercises in the Pilates repertoire, you need to stay healthy, active, and strong. Chapter 16 shows you the way.

Chapter 17 has special advice for people who are older or have a bad back or a stiff neck. If you fall into any of these categories, you may need to avoid certain exercises while focusing on others.

Chapter 16

Pilates for the Pregnant and Recently Pregnant

*P*regnancy is a time when a woman's body naturally puts on weight and grows in ways that make a healthy birth possible. An effective prenatal exercise program supports this natural process of expansion and addresses the potential weaknesses that arise during and after pregnancy that can leave a woman vulnerable to injury.

In this chapter, I provide an overview of what exercises are safe and important to do to support the extra weight and strain that pregnancy puts on your body. In addition, I offer general guidelines of what to avoid while pregnant.

Of course, after birth it's a whole different story. The body has completely different needs in the postnatal phase, and in this chapter I help you understand the concepts underlying the differences and hope to inspire you to maintain a regular and well-thought-out exercise program.

Prenatal Guidelines

If you were already doing Pilates for a while before you became pregnant, simply modify your program by following the guidelines and the protocol outlined in the following pages. Don't try to advance your level of Pilates exercises once you know you are pregnant — just stay at the same level, with some modifications. If you know a highly qualified Pilates instructor who has experience with training pregnant women, you will be safe doing Pilates at any time, as long as you follow the instructor's advice.

I usually tell people that they need to be very careful when *starting* a Pilates program when pregnant. If this is your first time doing Pilates and you are pregnant, please follow the guidelines in this book carefully, and you will gain the benefits of Pilates without fear of injury.

Keep the abs strong while the belly grows

Back pain is a common complaint of pregnant women as they get heavier and their bellies begin to protrude and put extra strain on their back. Keeping abdominal muscles strong during pregnancy is essential, because the abs support the extra weight and protect the back from injury and overstraining. But not all ab-strengthening exercises are created equal. You want to avoid *flexion* exercises and focus on stability exercises.

Flexion is the rounding of the spine forward when standing or sitting, or rolling upward when lying down. A sit-up is a type of flexion exercise. When doing a sit-up, the abdominal muscles are responsible for this action of flexion. A sit-up (which is a part of many Pilates exercises, including Upper Abdominal Curl, Roll Up, and Roll Down) compresses the abdomen and shortens the abdominal wall. This is *not* what you want to do when your belly is growing and expanding — as it is during pregnancy.

I believe it is not good to go against nature and attempt to contract that which should be expanding. Also, the superficial abdominal muscle (rectus abdominis) separates in some pregnant women, and I believe this problem can be exacerbated by sit-ups and anything that puts excessive compression on the abdomen.

Doing flexion exercises, which use the abdominal muscles, isn't a great idea if you're pregnant. In other words, sit-ups, in whatever form they take, are a no-no.

Instead of doing sit-ups, which load the abdomen, do exercises that strengthen the abdomen through stabilization instead of through flexion. Stabilization exercises work the deeper abdominal muscles, which are more important for supporting your back. Stabilization exercises involve working the deep abdominal muscles while keeping the torso stable. (For more about stabilization, see the section about the eight great principles in Chapter 1.)

In the pregnancy guidelines in this chapter, I basically took out all the sit-up-type exercises and left in all the other exercises that are beneficial to pregnant women.

Keep the rest of the body strong

Maintaining strength in your legs, hips, and upper body while you're pregnant is important, and not just to support the extra pounds you're carrying around now. You'll need the arm strength once the baby is born and you're picking up your not-so-little bundle of joy all the time. Plus, breast-feeding tends to pull you into a hunched-over position that can create discomfort in the upper back and shoulders. If you prepare your body for these challenges while you're pregnant, you're much less likely to injure yourself during and after the birth process, and you'll probably bounce back from the birth experience a lot faster. You can prepare yourself for postnatal life by maintaining a regular program of specific exercises — which I outline in this chapter — that incorporates both Pilates and non-Pilates exercises.

Don't overstretch

When a woman is pregnant, her body releases a chemical called elastin that relaxes the muscles, tendons, and ligaments to allow the baby to emerge through the pelvis. In other words, a woman who had tight muscles before pregnancy will notice a gradual loosening and an ability to go further in her stretches.

In the second and, especially, the third trimester, women need to be careful about doing stretches that go beyond their pre-pregnant range of motion. You can actually stretch too much and destabilize the joints — especially in the pelvic area. So while it's important that you keep the body open and stretched out to avoid muscle tension, it's equally important that you remain mindful of how far you are going in your stretches. The inner thigh is an especially vulnerable muscle that can negatively affect your pelvis if overstretched, so please don't go doing the Chinese splits just because suddenly you can!

Be moderate

I once heard that giving birth can burn more calories than running a marathon. Thus labor requires a tremendous amount of endurance, which is why exercising regularly during pregnancy is essential. Giving birth is the biggest workout of your life, and you need to be ready. Maintain a regular exercise program while pregnant, and be sure to include some gentle aerobic exercise like walking or swimming in addition to a stretching and strengthening method like Pilates or yoga. However, you need to be moderate in your approach.

Especially as you approach your third trimester, *moderation* is the key word to remember when you work out. Follow your intuition and don't overtax yourself or your baby. And if you are exercising regularly, eat enough to keep your baby very well-nourished and happy.

If you're already a serious athlete, modify your workouts — especially as you approach your second and third trimesters. Balance is essential in all areas of life, especially exercise. Excessive exercise during pregnancy can put strain on your body and take away energy and nourishment from the baby growing inside. I know a few obsessive athletes who danced, ran, and/or worked out for hours each day during their pregnancies, and they ended up having premature births or underweight babies.

Prenatal Exercises

In this section, I tell you what Pilates exercises are good to do when you're pregnant. I also give you a handful of new exercises.

Before I get into some specifics, here are some general guidelines for what to do when you're pregnant:

- ✔ Do stabilization exercises for the torso and hips.
- ✔ Keep your legs strong.
- ✔ Keep your arms and back strong.
- ✔ Stretch out your hips.
- ✔ Stretch out your back.

Keep these pointers in mind as to what *not* to do when pregnant:

- ✔ Don't do sit-ups.
- ✔ Don't do anything that feels like it is compressing the abdomen.
- ✔ Don't lie on your belly.
- ✔ Don't lie on your back in the third trimester. Doing so compresses the abdominal aorta and blocks blood flow to you and your baby.
- ✔ Don't stretch excessively during the second and third trimester.

Follow your instincts: If it doesn't feel good, don't do it!

Pilates exercises to do

You should know which specific Pilates exercises from this book are good to do. Here they are! You'll notice that some are part of the main series presented in Chapters 4, 5, 6, and 7. Some are from Chapters 8, 9, and 10, in which I suggest helpful add-ons to your routine. I provide the chapter number next to the name of each exercise.

Fundamentals

All of these fundamental exercises are done lying on your back, so do them only in the first and second trimester only.

- ✔ Shoulder Shrugs (Chapter 4)
- ✔ Shoulder Slaps (Chapter 4)
- ✔ Arm Reaches/Arm Circles (Chapter 4)
- ✔ Coccyx Curls (Chapter 4)
- ✔ Tiny Steps (Chapter 4)
- ✔ Rolling Like a Ball, Modified (Chapter 4)

Beginning exercises

- ✔ Bridge (first and second trimester only) (Chapter 5)
- ✔ Sexy Spine Stretch (Chapter 10)
- ✔ The Basic Cat (Chapter 10)
- ✔ Spine Stretch Forward (Chapter 5)

Intermediate exercises

- ✔ Open Leg Rocker (first and second trimester only) (Chapter 6)
- ✔ Mermaid (Chapter 10)
- ✔ The Seal (first and second trimester only) (Chapter 6)

Advanced exercises

- ✔ The Saw (Chapter 7)
- ✔ Shoulder Bridge (first and second trimester only) (Chapter 7)
- ✔ Side Bend/Advanced Mermaid (first and second trimester only) (Chapter 7)

✔ Spine Twist (Chapter 7)

✔ Control Front (first and second trimester only) (Chapter 7)

✔ Pilates Push-Up (first and second trimester only) (Chapter 7)

✔ Kneeling Side Kicks (first and second trimester only) (Chapter 7)

Super advanced exercises

✔ The Twist (first and second trimester only) (Chapter 8)

✔ The Star (first and second trimester only) (Chapter 8)

Side Kick Series

All the side kick exercises are safe and highly recommended throughout your whole pregnancy. See Chapter 9 for photos and descriptions.

Pilates-Kegel exercises

Pregnancy, labor, and birth put a whole lot of stretch and strain on the body, especially the pelvic floor muscles. Giving these muscles extra attention during pregnancy, as well as postnatally, is important. Kegel is the name of an exercise that is often prescribed to prenatal and postnatal women to tone up the pelvic floor muscles and to help prevent incontinence after birth. You can integrate Kegels into your Pilates workout and simultaneously tone the pelvic floor while working the abdominal muscles.

How do you do a Kegel? You can feel your pelvic floor muscles simply by squeezing the muscles you use when you have to hold your pee in. If you just imagine being at the grocery store, waiting in line to buy that pint of ice cream and jar of pickles and really needing to pee, then contract those muscles that keep you from peeing right in the store and you will be engaging the deep pelvic floor muscles.

Add this pelvic floor cue or Pilates Kegel to every exercise in your workout. Every time you initiate an exercise and think of pulling your navel in toward your spine, also think of your Kegel cue (holding your pee in). Also try adding in the extra cue of squeezing your anus and your vagina shut when doing this Pilates Kegel. (Doing so activates the posterior and anterior pelvic floor muscles, respectively.) Try holding the Kegel contraction throughout the exercise. The goal is to be able to hold the Kegel ultimately for two long breaths.

My sister, an obstetrician, prescribes Kegel exercises to her pregnant clients all the time. She recommends doing a set of ten Kegels, holding as long as you can each time, three times a day, increasing the length of each squeeze as you get stronger. All this Kegeling may seem tedious at first, but you (and your spouse) will enjoy the benefits later!

Spa therapy for the postnatal woman? Mais oui!

My friend who lives in the South of France told me that the French government paid for her postnatal Kegel lessons, as well as for a bunch of other special spa-type therapeutic pampering services to get the postnatal body back in shape. The French have the reputation of caring a lot about their sex lives and keeping their bodies feeling good — and they put government money behind that reputation. But you'll have to do that pampering yourself!

4 on the Floor

The 4 on the Floor exercises are great for strengthening your butt and legs. To begin, carefully get down on the floor so that that you are on your hands and knees. Align your hands underneath your shoulders and align your knees underneath your hips. Keep your neck long, focusing on the floor in front of you, as shown in Figure 16-1a. Next, do these four exercises in order.

1: Quadruped

The Quadruped is a classic back-rehabilitation exercise that builds core stabilization and strengthens the butt, back, and shoulder muscles. This exercise is especially useful for pregnant women because the starting position is on all fours, which is safe and comfortable throughout pregnancy. In addition, since you can't lie on your belly when pregnant, Quadruped can replace the prone exercises that strengthen the back and butt (like Swimming, the Swan, and so on) in your workout routine.

Inhale: Lift up the left arm and right leg, reaching them long away from each other (Figure 16-1b). Try to maintain absolute stability in the torso.

Exhale: Hold this position. Pull your stomach to the spine and squeeze your butt to help stabilize.

Switch sides and complete 6 repetitions, alternating sides.

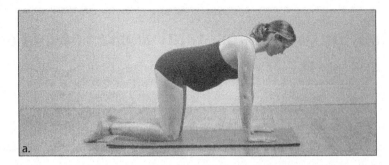

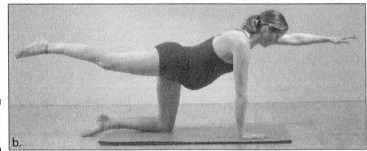

Figure 16-1:
Quadruped.

2: Single Leg Swimming on All Fours

Breathing continuously, lift up one leg and reach it long behind you, and pulse it up and down 10 times, keeping the torso stable and focusing on the butt doing the work (Figure 16-2).

Switch sides and complete 4 repetitions.

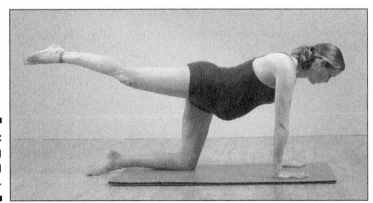

Figure 16-2:
Single Leg
Swimming
on All Fours.

3: Butt Cruncher on All Fours

Breathing continuously, lift up one leg and bend your knee so that the heel is toward the ceiling. Keep the hips square. Pulse the heel up and down 10 times, focusing on keeping the torso stable (Figure 16-3). Try not to arch the back.

Switch legs and do two sets of 10 with each leg.

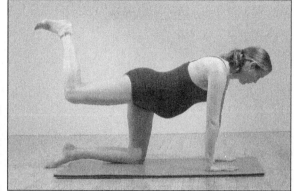

Figure 16-3: Butt Cruncher on All Fours.

4: Doggy Kicks on All Fours

Breathing continuously, lift up the right knee, keeping it bent at first, and bring it straight to the side, rotating open from the hip (Figure 16-4a). Then extend the right leg behind you, slightly diagonally to the right (Figure 16-4b). Keep the foot flexed and think of reaching long through your heel as if you're kicking someone diagonally behind you. Bring the leg back in to the bent position, then drop the knee back in line with the other leg to start again.

Complete 8 repetitions for each leg.

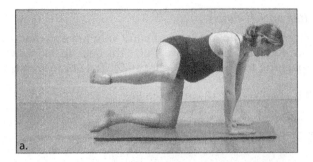

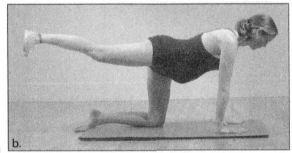

Figure 16-4:
Doggy Kicks
on All Fours.

Squats against the Wall with an Exercise Ball

Using an exercise ball to do Squats against the Wall gives you an excellent exercise for strengthening the thighs and butt. I go into more detail about the exercise ball in Chapter 13.

Getting set

Place the exercise ball behind your back against a wall. Start standing, leaning lightly into the ball. Your legs should be hip distance apart, a few feet in front of your torso, feet facing forward. Extend your arms out in front of you (Figure 16-5a).

The exercise

Slowly bend your knees, leaning some of your weight into the ball. Bend down only as far as you feel you can hold comfortably, never going lower than a 90-degree angle at the knee (Figure 16-5b). Keep your knees aligned over your middle toes, and think of pressing into your heels to engage the back of your legs and your butt. The ball should be in the small of your back, helping you maintain the Neutral Spine.

Hold for 2 breaths, circling your arms up and open for one breath, then reverse the arm circle for the second breath (Figure 16-5c). Slowly come back up. Complete 4 repetitions.

Modification

Do the same exercise, except start with your legs open twice as wide as your hips, turned out from the hips, knees facing away from each other (see Figure 16-6). Align your knees over your middle toes. Don't let your feet turn out more than your knees.

Hold for 2 breaths, circling your arms up and open for one breath, then reverse the arm circle for the second breath. Slowly come back up. Complete 4 repetitions.

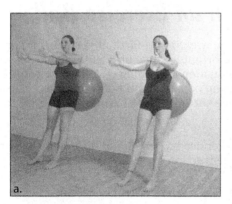

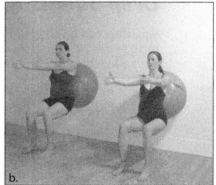

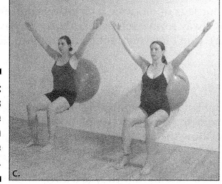

Figure 16-5:
Squats against the Wall with an Exercise Ball.

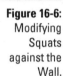

Figure 16-6:
Modifying
Squats
against the
Wall.

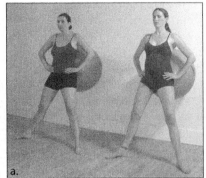 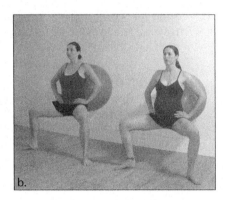

Deep Squats with an Exercise Ball

Squatting can be an ergonomic way to give birth. If you are thinking of giving birth in this position, it is important to open up your hip muscles and strengthen the legs. Even if you aren't planning on squatting while in labor, you will still benefit from having open hip and pelvic muscles. This exercise is great for this purpose. Make sure you have bare feet and good traction on the floor.

Some women actually have exercise balls on hand during birth. Lying and rolling on the ball is a great distraction from the pain, and you can relieve back strain while you're in labor.

Getting set

Sit on the exercise ball with your legs open twice as wide as your hips, turned out from the hips, knees facing away from each other. Align your knees over your middle toes (Figure 16-7a). Don't let your feet turn out more than your knees.

The exercise

Slowly bend your knees, leaning back, with your weight leaning into the ball as you walk your feet slowly away from you and come down into a deep squat (Figures 16-7b and 16-7c show this motion). (You can use your arms to support your weight on the ball as you walk down into your squat.) Allow your back to be molded around the ball and your pelvis dropped down as low as is comfortable. Adjust your feet so that they are aligned with the knees, and so that the whole foot is able to stay in contact with the floor.

Hold for 4 breaths, and slowly come back up. Complete 4 repetitions.

Modification

You can give your back a luxurious stretch. Starting from the deep squat position, begin to straighten your legs as you bring your arms up by your ears. Then reach back toward the ball behind you, guiding your body back so that your whole spine is stretched open on top of the ball. Let your head hang heavy on the ball, and breathe into this open back stretch. Slowly allow your arms to circle open, and as the arms complete the circle and start to come down by your sides, return to the deep squat position. Repeat three times. Hold the squat position each time for a few breaths to strengthen the legs and open up the hips. Figure 16-8 shows the modification.

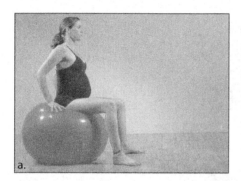
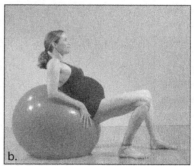

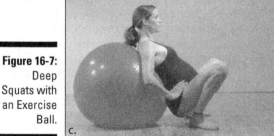

Figure 16-7: Deep Squats with an Exercise Ball.

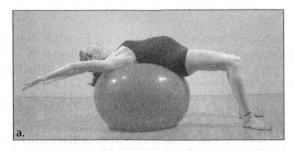

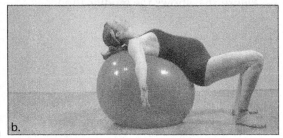

Figure 16-8:
Modifying
Deep
Squats to
get a great
stretch.

Postnatal Guidelines

Mothers need to be strong! Caring for a new baby puts many hidden strains on the body. Picking up a child, holding a child on your hip, breast-feeding, and simply getting up and down from bed can be hard on your body, especially your back. Pilates is the perfect exercise technique for the postnatal woman. Of course, finding time to take care of yourself is the hardest part of all for a new mother. But if you do 10 to 20 minutes a day, you will feel a big difference. I don't know of anything better to get your body back in shape than Pilates.

After birth, the abdominal muscles are very stretched out and have little tone. This lack of muscle tone can make a woman vulnerable to back injury, especially given the physical taxations of a new mother. If you have been doing a consistent Pilates program during pregnancy, your abdominal muscle tone will bounce back at a much faster rate than it otherwise would. If you haven't been doing Pilates, this is a great time to start! The great thing about being a mom instead of being a pregnant woman is that you don't have to worry so much about what not to do.

All Pilates exercises are great for the postnatal woman, just make sure you have given yourself adequate time to heal from birth. Follow your doctor's recommendations on that count. Start with the fundamentals and slowly work your way up, just like everyone else, except that you should have a little more patience with yourself.

If you're breastfeeding, I particularly recommend the basic shoulder set from Chapter 11, done with the roller. The roller is great at countering the upper back and neck strain caused by breastfeeding.

Special advice if you've had a cesarean

If you've had a cesarean, your doctor has probably told you not to do anything that will put strain on your abdominals for six weeks, until the scar has healed. This includes lifting heavy objects. Once you're ready to begin strengthening your belly, don't be surprised if you have trouble feeling your abdominal muscles at first. Like after any abdominal surgery, you must realize that all your abdominal muscles have been cut straight through, and scar tissue has replaced normal muscle tissue. You must have patience with yourself.

Start with the stabilizing abdominal exercises. Don't do sit-ups at first, but instead try to find your deep Abdominal Scoop while keeping your torso stable. You may not feel your full strength in your belly again for at least a year; this is not unusual. Some people will bounce back easier than others. Try the cesarean program for four weeks before moving on to the regular Pilates mat work series. Listen to your body; if you don't feel ready to move on, keep doing this program as long as you need to.

I highly recommend that you buy yourself a small ball to help you find your deep abdominals (see Chapter 12). Here's the cesarean program to get you started.

- ✔ Deep Abdominal Cue with small ball (Chapter 12)
- ✔ Coccyx Curls (Chapter 4)
- ✔ Tiny Steps (Chapter 4)
- ✔ Bridge (Chapter 4)
- ✔ Single Leg Bridge (Chapter 5)
- ✔ Side Kicks (Chapter 9)
- ✔ The Basic Cat (Chapter 10)
- ✔ Quadruped (This Chapter)

Chapter 17

Special Routines for Special Situations

Not all Pilates exercises are good for everyone. If you're over 60 years old, suffer from neck and shoulder tension, or have lower back pain, then read on. You may need a special Pilates program.

In the medical profession, the first rule is always "Do no harm." If you have any kind of special health issue, having some knowledge of what *not* to do is important so that your issue doesn't become even more of an issue. See Chapter 4 for more signs that an exercise isn't right for you.

Benefiting from Pilates If You're Older

Being over 60 doesn't have to be a health issue, but you do need to take some precautions when beginning a new exercise program. I'm in my late 30s, and have been active most of my life. I've suffered a few serious injuries over the years, but all in all I feel that my body is still able to do most of what I want it to. I have noticed, however, that in the last few years I must be much more careful about warming up before attempting super fantastic tricks. I can't just wake up and do a back flip anymore, but must painstakingly go through the rigmarole of getting my muscles warm and my joints juicy.

Don't think that I'm complaining! My point is that as we get older, we must acknowledge the natural changes in our physiques, and we must spend more time preparing the body for the challenges of exercise. The bones become more calcified and brittle, the muscles lose their elasticity, and the protective structures around the joints lose their fluid. All these changes increase the potential for impact and injury. Certain types of movement exacerbate the wear and tear on the skeleton and soft tissues. In this section, you find out which movements to avoid and what types of exercises promote longevity of the body and increase the body's ability to move freely.

One of the most common symptoms of aging is loss of flexibility in the spine. This loss of flexibility can be reversed by doing . . . guess what . . . Pilates!

Always see your doctor before starting any new exercise program. And I'm not just saying this because of the lawyers. Your doctor knows your medical history and may be aware of reasons why you shouldn't do Pilates.

Exercises you may want to avoid

Do the following exercises with caution. If you feel fine doing them, then go right ahead!

- These exercises have you roll onto your neck:
    - Hip-Up (Chapter 4)
    - Rolling Like a Ball (Chapters 4 and 5)
    - Rollover (Chapter 7)
    - Jackknife (Chapter 7)
    - Super Advanced Corkscrew (Chapter 8)
    - Open Leg Rocker (Chapter 6)
    - Seal (Chapter 6)
- These exercises call for dramatic extension of the spine:
    - The high part of Rising Swan (Chapter 5)
    - Swan Dive (Chapter 8)
- Rounding your back forward while bearing weights can hurt your back, so consider omitting the free weights when Rolling Down the Wall (Chapter 14).

Exercises you may want to focus on

If you're new to Pilates, start with Chapter 4 like everyone else, after you've read the first three chapters, especially Chapter 3. After that, go carefully with anything that doesn't feel good to you. Here are some pretty good bets.

✔ To strengthen your abdominal muscles, do the following:

- • Upper Abdominal Curls (Chapter 4, 12, and 13 have versions)
- • Hundred (Chapters 5, 6, and 7 have versions)
- • The Fives (see the sidebar in Chapter 6)

✔ To strengthen your back, do the following:

- • Single Leg Kick (Chapter 6)
- • Double Leg Kick (Chapter 6)

✔ To strengthen your butt, do the Side Kick series in Chapter 9.

✔ To be better able to stabilize your torso, do the following:

- • Tiny Steps (Chapter 4 on the mat and Chapter 11 with a roller)
- • Arm Reaches/Arm Circles (Chapter 4 on the mat and Chapter 11 with a roller)
- • Bridge and the single leg variation of Bridge (Chapter 5 on the mat and Chapter 13 with the big ball. Chapter 12 also has the Bridge with the small ball, but there's no single-leg variation)
- • Quadruped (Chapter 16)

✔ To stretch your back, do the following:

- • The Cat Stretches (Chapter 10). You may need to put some padding under your knees if kneeling hurts.
- • Coccyx Curls (Chapter 4)
- • Mermaid (Chapter 10). You may need to sit on a pillow.

✔ To stretch your shoulders, do the basic shoulder set (Chapter 11) on the roller.

Reducing Pain in Your Neck and Shoulders

Tension in the neck and shoulders is one of the most common health complaints of the modern age. People tend to sit at a computer for hours at a time. Even at the most ergonomic workstation, overtaxing the neck and shoulder muscles is almost impossible to avoid. Being so sedentary isn't natural, and it's really straining on your shoulder muscles to hold your arms in front of you for hours at a time as you type. People also tend to hold emotional tension and stress in their necks. Pilates exercises can help you relax those muscles. I have one word for neck and shoulder tension: roller (see Chapter 11). Using the roller is one of the most effective ways to reduce tension in the upper body.

✔ To release the neck and shoulder muscles, try the following:

- Shoulder Shrugs (Chapter 4)

- Shoulder Slaps (Chapter 4 on the mat and Chapter 11 with a roller)

- Arm Reaches/Arm Circles (Chapter 4 on the mat and Chapter 11 with a roller)

- Chicken Wings (on the roller, Chapter 11)

- Angels in the Snow (on the roller, Chapter 11)

- Open Back Stretch (on the big ball, Chapter 13)

- Rolling Down the Wall (Chapter 14)

✔ To strengthen the deep neck muscles, do these exercises:

- Upper Abdominal Curls (Chapter 4)

- Rising Swan (Chapter 5 on the mat)

- The Swan (Chapter 11 on the roller)

- Arm Circles on the Wall (Chapter 14)

- Chicken Wings on the Wall (a modification of Arm Circles on the Wall in Chapter 14)

Easing Your Back Pain with Pilates

I said it before, and I'll say it again. Most back pain is due to faulty posture. And when I say faulty posture, I mean the posture in which you spend most of your days.

Do you sit at a desk and stare straight ahead? Unfortunately, many people do, and they find it very difficult to sit up with proper posture for eight hours at a time. It becomes a vicious cycle: First you sit for long periods of time in a way that doesn't properly support the spine (generally, in a slightly hunched-over position). Then you lose strength in your postural muscles by not using them day after day, and then you can't sit up properly even if you wanted to because you've lost strength! What to do? I mean, besides quitting your day job and joining the circus? Well guess what? Pilates! Once again, Pilates can save the day.

Most of the Pilates mat exercises strengthen the muscles necessary to properly support the spine and bring an awareness about what proper posture actually is. It's not enough just to do Pilates mat exercises; if you want to improve your posture and heal your back pain, you must incorporate Pilates into your daily life. You must translate the Neutral Spine, the feeling of length, and the Abdominal Scoop into your desk job. If you can incorporate the deeper Pilates concepts into your daily life, you'll notice changes immediately — in your back pain, in your posture, and in your sense of well-being.

Understanding the common causes of lower back pain

Again, most back pain is a result of bad posture when sitting, standing, or walking. The main things to remember to prevent bad posture are to sit and stand up tall, keep your belly pulled in, and keep your shoulder blades pulling down your back. When you find your correct posture, you should feel the ease it creates in your whole back.

You may need to slowly work up to sitting properly for long periods of time. Even your postural muscles need to get in shape. But the more awareness you have, the better you will feel. If you stand a lot, think of keeping your knees soft; don't lock them. Try to keep even weight on both legs. Keep your belly pulled in.

But bad posture isn't the only culprit. A sedentary lifestyle is also often to blame. Let's face it: We weren't meant to sit at a computer monitor for eight hours a day — or to sit on a chair at all, for that matter. Sitting isn't easy on your back. If you think about it, when you sit in a chair, the back muscles have to work all the time to keep you upright. Your legs are not able to help out at all. Furthermore, staying in one position doesn't promote good circulation and muscle tone. Break up your work day by getting up regularly from your chair and stretching out, going for a walk, or doing a Pilates series, if you can.

Avoiding loaded flexion

Most construction workers have terrible backs by the time they're 40, because they spend much of their day bending over and lifting up heavy objects. Even if you maintain perfect alignment when lifting, you can't avoid loading the spine in flexion if you're installing a floor, say, or doing much of anything below the waist.

Flexion is the rounding forward of the spine when standing or sitting, or what your spine does when rolling up in a sit-up. *Loaded* means . . . well, loaded. An example of loading the spine in flexion is the Rolling Down the Wall exercise from Chapter 14 if you have free weights in your hands. As you roll forward, the weight of your head, body, and the free weights is dropping down. The muscles and ligaments of the back are supporting that weight. Another example of loaded flexion is the Hip-Up exercise. As you lift your hips, the weight of the butt and legs is now on your back. If you roll back too far, the weight of your whole body will be on your neck. The neck is especially vulnerable to having too much load because it is made up of small, fragile vertebrae that are not meant to hold up anything but your head when standing. When you get very strong in your core, your spine can support more weight without being traumatized.

Flexion is the movement of the spine that most damages the structures of the spine, especially the intervertebral discs and the ligaments of the back. If you feel uncomfortable when doing flexion exercises, don't do them! Instead, do all the exercises that don't bother your back, and come back to the others when you have more strength.

To avoid loaded flexion, use proper body mechanics when bending over and lifting:

- Keep Neutral Spine. You can just think of keeping the spine straight. Don't round the back forward (flexion).

- Bend your knees; and if you're lifting something, use your leg muscles, not your back!

- Keep your Abdominal Scoop by pulling your navel in toward your spine. Doing so helps support the back.

Being your own guide

A well-known doctor named Robin McKenzie wrote a book called *Treat Your Own Back,* which revolutionized the way the rehabilitation profession viewed back pain. Basically, the book describes a program in which you experiment and find out what movements exacerbate your back pain, and what movements and positions alleviate your back pain. Then you do the things that make you feel better. It sounds so fabulously simple, and it works. I agree with this approach and suggest that you follow the same principles when doing Pilates.

Let pain be your guide, not your nemesis. When trying a new exercise, see if the movement makes your back pain worse or better. Use this information to heal yourself. For instance, if you find that flexion (rounding the spine forward), as in Spine Stretch Forward, makes your back feel great, then you can proceed with all the flexion exercises with a fair bit of confidence. In that case, exercises that do the opposite movement, extension (arching the back), as in the Rising Swan, may make your back hurt. If this is so, avoid all exercises that extend the back. The act of twisting may be the source of the problem, or it could be twisting in just one direction. Take note of what hurts and apply this information to your workout.

When you're in pain, you must be very mindful when trying out new exercises. I recommend seeing a doctor first to make sure you don't have any serious injury, and then going to a Pilates instructor trained in rehabilitation if you are worried about hurting yourself.

Exercises you may want to avoid

If you have lower back pain, you may want to follow these guidelines:

- ✔ Proceed with caution when doing any exercise that involves loaded flexion, but also remember that some people feel relief by doing flexion exercises. If you're one of those people, don't worry too much about the following list.

  - Hip-Up (Chapter 4)
  - Rolling Like a Ball (Chapters 4 and 5)
  - Rollover (Chapter 7)
  - Jackknife (Chapter 7)
  - Super Advanced Corkscrew (Chapter 8)
  - Open Leg Rocker (Chapter 6)
  - Seal (Chapter 6)

- ✔ Be leery of these exercises that involve drastic extension of the spine:

  - Rising Swan (Chapter 5)
  - Swan Dive (Chapter 8)

- ✔ You may want to avoid rounding forward with excessive weight, as in the Rolling Down the Wall with free weights (Chapter 14).

Exercises you may want to focus on

Every individual is different — or more to the point, every *back* is different. But here are some exercises that you very well may find doable and that may alleviate your pain:

- ✔ To stretch the back, try these exercises:

  - The Cat Stretches (Chapter 10)
  - Coccyx Curls (Chapter 4)
  - Mermaid (Chapter 10)

- ✔ To strengthen the thighs and butt, do the Side Kick series (Chapter 9).

- ✔ To improve your ability to stabilize your torso, give these a try:

  - Tiny Steps (Chapter 4 and, with a roller, Chapter 11)
  - Arm Reaches/Arm Circles (Chapter 4 and, with a roller, Chapter 11)
  - Bridge and single leg variation (Chapter 5)
  - Quadruped (even if you're not pregnant) (Chapter 16)

✔ To stretch your hips and legs, do these exercises:

- Hamstring Stretch (described as part of the Scissors exercise in Chapter 6)

- Hip Flexor Stretch (Chapter 7)

✔ To stretch your back, try all the exercises in Chapter 10 (but watch out for Sexy Spine Stretch because of the twisting aspect — this can exacerbate some back problems).

Part V
The Part of Tens

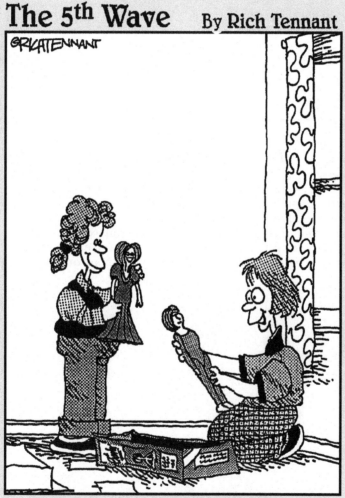

The 5th Wave   By Rich Tennant

"...and this one's Pilates Barbie. She doesn't come with a lot of stuff, but she can do the Boomerang without breaking."

In this part . . .

Every *For Dummies* book ends with easy-to-read chapters that have top ten lists. In this part, you find out what I think are the ten most important exercises, and why; you read about ten changes you can expect to see if you stick with Pilates; and you discover ten easy ways to incorporate Pilates into your daily life, among other things.

Chapter 18

The Ten Most Important Exercises

Determining the top ten Pilates exercises isn't easy because different exercises are good for different people. Yet, some exercises seem to stand out as the best exercises. If you were to poll a hundred Pilates instructors, each one would probably come up with a different ten, and each would have a valid reason. This chapter highlights my own Pilates picks and offers details on why they are so effective.

Coccyx Curls

Neither Coccyx Curls nor Upper Abdominal Curls are actually part of the classic Pilates repertoire, but are considered pre-Pilates exercises (Chapter 4). I consider these two to be essential for warming up the spine before attempting the Hundred, which is the classic Pilates first exercise. I start every workout with Coccyx Curls, no matter how advanced the workout. Why? Three reasons:

Coccyx Curls

✔ Warm up the lower back.

✔ Get you scooping. This exercise gets you in touch with your deep abdominals.

✔ Get you connected with your butt and hamstrings.

Upper Abdominal Curls

Upper Abdominal Curls (Chapter 4) are the second exercise I do with everyone, right after Coccyx Curls.

Upper Abdominal Curls

- ✔ Warm up the upper back and neck.

- ✔ Strengthen your upper abdominals, while developing stability in Neutral Spine in the lower back and pelvis.

- ✔ Teach proper neck alignment. When you lift your head off the mat and think of squeezing a tangerine under your chin, you are using your deep neck muscles, which are important for neck health.

Hundred

Hundred (Chapters 5, 6, and 7) is the first exercise in the classic Pilates repertoire. If your body and spine are warm before hitting the mat, Hundred is a fine way to start your mat routine. But if you're not warm, or it is in the morning and you're still stiff, I think starting with the Hundred puts too much stretch on the neck to begin a workout. That is why I recommend Coccyx Curls and Upper Abdominal Curls to start. But after you warm up, Hundred is an excellent exercise for the following three reasons:

Hundred

- ✔ Is a great way to get you really warm and maybe a bit sweaty.

- ✔ Is one of the best exercises to connect the breath to the abdominal muscles using percussive breathing.

- ✔ Strengthens the deep abdominals and neck muscles.

Bridge

Everyone can do Bridge (Chapter 5) safely: the young, the old, and the restless. The three reasons this exercise makes the top ten:

Bridge

- ✔ Teaches torso stability.

- ✔ Strengthens the butt and back of the legs (the gluteus maximus and hamstrings).

- ✔ The single leg variation improves lower back and pelvic stability (by working the gluteus medius).

Roll Down and Roll Up

Roll Down (Chapter 5) is the beginning version of the Roll Up (Chapter 6). This very basic exercise uses your whole abdominal wall and helps you in daily life. (Think how many times in your life you need to get up from lying down!)

Roll Down/Roll Up

- ✔ Strengthens abdominals.
- ✔ Strengthens hip flexors (psoas).
- ✔ Stretches the spine.

Rolling Like a Ball

Rolling Like a Ball (Chapters 4 and 5) is fun and good for you. I always feel like a little girl when I do this exercise. The three reasons this exercise makes the top ten:

Rolling Like a Ball

- ✔ Increases back flexibility.
- ✔ Massages the back.
- ✔ Teaches control from the deep abdominals.

Rising Swan

The Rising Swan (Chapter 5) is a lovely exercise. The three reasons this exercise makes the top ten:

Rising Swan

- ✔ Strengthens back and neck muscles and reverses the effects of slumping.
- ✔ Stretches the chest and abdominal muscles.
- ✔ Strengthens butt and hamstring muscles when done correctly.

Side Kicks

I love the Side Kick series (Chapter 9) because it can really work the butt. The three reasons this series makes the top ten:

Side Kicks

- ✔ Strengthen butt muscles (gluteus maximus and medius).
- ✔ Build torso stability.
- ✔ Are doable even if you're pregnant.

Swimming

Swimming (Chapter 7) is a full-body exercise that has many benefits. The three reasons it makes the top ten:

Swimming

- ✔ Strengthens the back and neck muscles.
- ✔ Trains proper neck alignment.
- ✔ Reverses the effects of slumping.

Sexy Spine Stretch

Sometimes I believe that the Sexy Spine Stretch (Chapter 10) is like a self-adjustment for the spine. You may even hear a popping noise like when you get adjusted at the chiropractor. This sound is the spine realigning. The three reasons this exercise makes the top ten:

Sexy Spine Stretch

- ✔ Works the spine and back muscles.
- ✔ Works your chest and pectoral muscles.
- ✔ Makes your spine twist, thereby increasing flexibility.

Chapter 19

Ten Changes You Can Expect to See from Pilates

In This Chapter

▶ Discovering how your body can change from doing Pilates

▶ Knowing what to expect from all the sweat and toil

*T*his chapter is meant to get you excited about starting your Pilates program. You won't see these changes immediately. Some of the changes you may not notice until three months into your Pilates workouts. Be patient. No exercise program works miracles, but I still maintain that Pilates is magic.

These changes in your body become apparent only if you maintain a regular Pilates program, meaning doing the workout at least twice a week.

A Firmer Butt

Most of the Pilates exercises in this book somehow or other work the butt. You should notice a definite change within a few weeks of doing Pilates regularly. Your butt should be more toned and perhaps a little smaller. If you start with a very small and undeveloped butt, it actually may grow a little, but in a very nice way.

Longer and Leaner Musculature

A ballet dancer was rejected from a ballet company because her body was too bulky and her "line wasn't ideal." This dancer did Pilates for a year and reauditioned, and is now the principal dancer in this same company. Why? Because Pilates transformed this dancer's body to a more ideal shape. She started out with big hulking thighs that were strong but just too big to look perfect in a tutu. After doing Pilates for a year, her thighs got longer and leaner but still had the strength and flexibility required of a professional dancer.

If you are like this ballet dancer, and tend to bulk up when you work out, Pilates is an ideal strength-training program for you. Pilates exercises accentuate the length of the limbs and change bulky muscles into longer and leaner ones. For more details about this side effect of Pilates, see Chapter 2. In general, Pilates exercise should lengthen your muscles and make you look taller.

Better Posture

Better posture is something I can pretty much guarantee. And other people will surely notice this change in you after only a few Pilates workouts. If you take the lessons you learn from Pilates to heart, you'll stand and sit taller and look more elegant. In Figure 19-1, the model is standing in a classic Pilates posture. Remember, this position isn't natural for everyone, and frankly, I don't recommend standing exactly like her. She's standing with her legs turned out, which isn't the most natural position unless you're taking a ballet class. But she does demonstrate some important rules about posture that everyone should be aware of when standing:

✔ Pull your navel in toward your spine.

✔ Keep your head balanced on top of your hips (not forward or behind).

✔ Lengthen the back of your neck.

✔ Keep your shoulders back and down and keep your back wide.

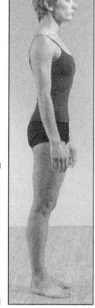

Figure 19-1:
Good posture — although this position may not be natural for everyone.

Forward head posture

Forward head posture, as shown in Figure 19-2, is very common for humans who live on planet Earth. The tendency to jut our heads forward is a natural side effect of having your eyes in the front of your head. When you sit at a desk and look at a computer or study a book, you tend to let your head go forward of your body. Proper ergonomics can help reduce this tendency, but won't completely alleviate the gravitational pull of the head forward. Pilates is a great antidote for this posture problem. Pilates exercises are almost always aimed at aligning the spine so that the head sits on top of the hips, not in front. If you imagine you have a golden string attached to the back of the top of your head, and it's pulling you up toward the heavens, you'll naturally correct your forward head posture.

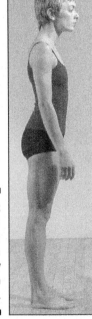

Figure 19-2:
Forward
head
posture, a
very
common
problem.

Uptight posture

The upper trapezius muscles are workaholics. The "traps" are those muscles at the top of your shoulders and at the back of your neck that always could use a nice massage. These muscles love to hold tension. It's like they enjoy being tight and think they can just hold up the world. Actually, desk work and computer work are the main culprits that exacerbate neck and shoulder tension. Pilates addresses this problem in the very first exercise in Chapter 4, Shoulder Shrugs. Once you become aware of the tension that is constantly present in these muscles, you can begin to consciously release tension. Pilates teaches you how to relax the traps and at the same time engage the opposing muscles to keep the traps happy and tension-free. Figure 19-3 shows uptight posture.

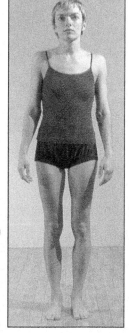

Figure 19-3:
Feeling
tense?
Uptight
posture.

Poochy belly posture

Some people just have a poochy belly. Maybe their mothers never told them to suck in their gut. Or maybe they've given birth recently. Or maybe they drink too many beers. Or maybe they just don't think of pulling their navel in to their spine. If that's the case, one session with me and the pooch is gone. The first thing I teach someone is the Abdominal Scoop, and you'd be surprised how much difference this small idea can have on a person's body. You can decrease your waist by a good three inches just by using your deep abdominals and pulling your belly in toward your spine. Try it! If you practice Pilates regularly, over time your belly will naturally be flatter without your having to always think about it. Figure 19-4 shows poochy belly posture.

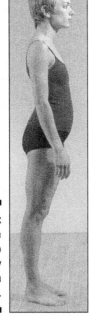

Figure 19-4:
Make the pooch go away by sucking in your gut.

A Flatter Tummy

The best way to get a flatter tummy is to lose a little weight. The second best way is to do Pilates. If you're already thin but have a bulge in your middle, Pilates can help you lose a notch in your belt. The most basic aspect of the Pilates method is pulling your navel in toward your spine or scooping your abdominals. If you apply this simple technique to your everyday life — when standing, walking, and so on — your belly will be flatter and more attractive.

Less Back Pain

Most back pain results from faulty posture and a sedentary lifestyle. Pilates addresses the muscle imbalances that most typically contribute to back pain, namely weak abdominals and butt muscles. Pilates also stretches out the tight and overworked back muscles.

Proper alignment is the main factor that helps to alleviate back pain. If you do Pilates carefully, you'll understand how to use your body in ways that protect your back from injury. Pilates is one of the best methods to use to keep your back healthy, no matter what your age or vocation, or what other exercise regimens you may do. For more information about Pilates and back pain, refer to Chapter 17.

More Flexibility

Pilates exercises stretch the muscles and the joints while they strengthen the body. If you have found that your spine has lost some of its range of motion and flexibility, Pilates very quickly lessens this problem. Everyone has physical limitations that depend on age, genetics, and lifestyle. Pilates is not a panacea, but if you do a regular Pilates exercise program, your body can reach its potential in the areas of flexibility and strength.

Better Sex

Pilates brings about a newfound body control that affects all aspects of life, including sex. You may find that, because of increased back and hip flexibility, you can get into positions that previously had been impossible. You may also discover increased control of your pelvic muscles, thereby enhancing sexual pleasure (see Chapter 16). If having sex hurts your back, you may find that you're going to love what Pilates can do for you! And so will your partner.

More Awareness

If nothing else, doing Pilates should give you a new awareness of your body. You may never have thought about pulling in your tummy, sitting up tall, or keeping your shoulder blades down away from your ears. And you may never have thought a lot about how you breathe. The things you find out in Pilates will start to filter into your daily life, and you may find that you correct your own posture and habits naturally.

Better Balance

Any gymnast knows that to keep from falling off the balance beam, you need to pull in your belly and squeeze your butt. I learned this concept from "Mr. T," my high school gymnastics coach, who always reminded me while on the balance beam to "squeeze that silver dollar." (You can imagine where that silver dollar was located.) He knew nothing of Pilates, but the same concepts apply. In order to have good balance, you need to have a strong center, and you need to know how to find it without a lot of thought. Pilates exercises strengthen the core. After doing Pilates regularly, you may not be able to do a back flip on the balance beam, but you'll definitely find increased coordination and balance.

Greater Strength

Any exercise regimen should increase your body's overall strength, or else what's the point? But Pilates strengthens the muscles in your body that you may actually notice on a day-to-day basis. Pilates is meant to improve your daily life: It can help you get up from bed, if that's hard for you, or it can help you do a triple back flip off the diving board, if that's your goal. Whatever activity you do, you'll find that Pilates exercises improve strength in meaningful ways and can help with the overall health of your spine. Doing Pilates can prevent injuries, too!

Chapter 20

Ten Simple Ways to Incorporate Pilates into Your Everyday Life

*E*ven if you were to do Pilates for an hour every day, you wouldn't get the profound results that Pilates has to offer if you reverted to bad postural habits for the rest of your day. Some people naturally take what they learn from Pilates and bring it to their non-Pilates activities, while others find it hard to break old habits. In this chapter, you discover concrete ways to improve your posture, help your back pain, and achieve a general sense of well-being.

Doing Pilates and improving your posture go hand in hand. Anything you can do away from the mat or Pilates studio to improve your posture is a continuation of your Pilates experience.

Do the Basic Cat Stretch Every Morning

If you were a cat, you'd do the Basic Cat every morning without even thinking about it. If you have a pet, you've probably noticed that it always stretches out its spine after a nap or a long rest in the sun. I recommend starting your day with a spine stretch to get the blood circulating and to get the kinks out before starting your day. The Basic Cat is a particularly good stretch for the morning because it's very safe and gentle and doesn't put unnecessary strain on a stiff spine. See Chapter 10 for details about the Basic Cat.

Think of a Golden String Pulling You Up from the Back of the Top of Your Head

Holding an image in your head can help you change your body dramatically. Working out with a regular Pilates routine does wonders, but thinking about proper alignment for the rest of your day does even more. Try to remember to stand up with the back of the top of your head pulled up toward the sky, thereby lengthening your spine.

Keep Your Belly Scoop Whenever You Can

Pulling your navel in toward your spine protects your back from potential injury. Using your deep abdominals, especially when bending over and lifting, takes some of the strain off your back. The more you practice sucking in your gut, the stronger your deep abdominals become and the easier it is to keep that belly flat.

Keep Your Shoulders Relaxed and Pulling Down Your Back

It's easy to unconsciously hunch your shoulders. This is one of the most common misuses of muscles, and working at a desk or computer exacerbates this tendency. Relax your shoulders, and keep pulling the shoulder blades down and away from your ears. Think of using the muscles underneath the shoulder blades to keep the shoulders in their proper dropped position. Doing so works wonders for your neck!

Remember to Breathe Deeply

Take a moment each day to breathe deeply and slowly. Most people use only about half of their lung capacity. Try to take a breath that fills up the lowest portion of your lungs. This style of breathing is relaxing and good for your health. Lungs are three-dimensional and extend as far back as your ribs go. Breathing wide into the ribs, instead of up and down, can actually stretch the back and release muscle tension.

Get a Lumbar Support Pillow for Work and Your Car

A lumbar pillow supports your lower back and helps you maintain Neutral Spine while you work and drive. Remember that improper posture is the number one reason for back pain. You can buy a lumbar support at most large drugstores, variety stores, or back care stores. You simply place it in the small of your back and, *voilà*, you can feel your posture improving effortlessly!

Sit Up Tall when Working

If you don't have a lumbar support pillow, then you must support your back all by yourself. You can do so just by thinking the right thoughts. I can't say this enough; most back pain is due to faulty posture and sitting incorrectly. Please sit up tall, trying to lift up from the lower back, so that you have Neutral Spine when sitting. Your head should be balanced in a straight line on top of your hips, not jutting out in front.

Sit on a Big Ball at Work

I know you might feel silly, but if you can manage it at your workplace, try sitting on a fitness ball instead of a chair for some of your work day. You might discover that sitting on a ball is a savior for your back, especially if you find sitting on a chair for long periods of time uncomfortable. Sitting on a ball forces you to sit up tall while keeping the natural curves of the spine. Slouching is almost impossible, so the postural muscles of your back become stronger. Over time, you'll be able to sit on the ball for longer and longer periods of time.

Sitting without a chair to support your spine requires a strong back, so try sitting on the ball only part of the time. In addition, you can periodically stretch out your back on the ball (see Open Back Stretch in Chapter 13).

Get a Cervical Pillow for Your Bed

A cervical pillow (or neck pillow) looks like an oversized hot dog and goes behind your neck when you're lying on your back or on your side. The pillow functions to support the natural curve of your neck.

Chronic neck soreness often results from an improper sleeping position. This type of pillow is especially useful if you wake up with neck pain.

You can experiment by rolling up a towel in the shape of a hot dog and putting it behind your neck. See if it helps before investing in the real thing.

Everyone has a favorite position that they like to sleep in. Some are better than others for your neck:

- ✔ Sleeping on your back puts the least strain on your neck.

- ✔ Sleeping on your side is the next best position, but make sure that you have support under the curve of your neck and also make sure that your pillow is not so big that it's tilting your head upward. You want to sleep in a neutral position for your neck, supporting its natural curve.

- ✔ Sleeping on your belly is the worst for your neck, because your neck is in a very strained position. If you sleep on your belly, you may actually injure your neck while you sleep.

Walk the Right Way

Imagine that you're a supermodel on a catwalk. When you stride down the street, think of walking with a long stride, initiating the movement from the hips and butt, not just the knees. This way of walking increases the length of your stride while stretching out the front of your hips (your hip flexors). Walking with long strides helps reverse the tightness in the hips and back that comes from long bouts of sitting.

Chapter 21

Ten Questions to Ask When Choosing a Studio or Instructor

*T*his chapter is meant to help you choose a good Pilates studio and find a competent instructor. Find out the answers to these questions before you decide where to do your Pilates workout.

You can have a completely satisfying Pilates experience in your own home, with nothing but a mat and this book. But if you live in an area where you can find a Pilates studio, think about taking a class or getting individual instruction to give your workouts a boost.

Is Your Instructor Certified?

Many people around the country teach Pilates without completing a certification program. Such a program may or may not guarantee the skill of your instructor, but you can rest assured that someone who goes through a rigorous training program actually has something valuable to offer.

Many teachers work at my studio while they're *in the process* of getting certified. I think this arrangement is fine. They're in the process of accumulating hours and have already completed hundreds of hours of theoretical and practical Pilates education. They're also under the tutelage of an experienced instructor so they can continue to hone their skills. The ones to worry about are those who have never enrolled in an official course or those who dropped out and never completed their hours and their testing.

When Pilates instructors don't know their stuff, the potential for injury in their classes is increased, just as it would be in any exercise class taught by someone without the necessary credentials.

How Many Hours Was the Certification Course?

Unlike medicine, acupuncture, massage, and chiropractic, Pilates is an unregulated industry, meaning that there is no certifying board to set a standard of practice. Certification programs range from weekend-long mat certifications to two-year intensive courses. The general rule is that a good certification course includes a minimum 600 hours of total training, requiring at least a year to complete. Anything less is just not good enough for you and your body. Feel free to inquire about the depth of your trainer's knowledge and education before starting any Pilates instruction.

How Long Has Your Instructor Been Teaching?

The longer someone's been teaching Pilates, the more knowledge and experience she has, just like in any profession. You'll definitely notice the difference between a newly certified trainer and one who has been working with people's bodies for many years. If the price is the same, go for the most experienced trainer you can find.

Is Your Instructor Trained in Rehabilitation?

If you're not injured and want a workout, then you need to ask a different question: Does your instructor give a challenging workout? Skip this section and go to the next one.

Certain teacher-training programs focus mainly on fitness, while others stress alignment and injury rehabilitation. Many Pilates instructors complete additional training programs and devote their careers to working with people who have acute and chronic injuries. For instance, several rehabilitation specialists in my studio have gone through a separate rehabilitation workshop in addition to their Pilates certification. So if you are injured and want to use Pilates to help you recover, find an instructor who focuses on Pilates for rehabilitation.

Does Your Instructor Give a Challenging Workout?

Not all Pilates trainers are created equal. Some Pilates trainers give you a challenging workout, and some don't. Certain schools of Pilates are very fitness oriented and focus on muscular conditioning, and others focus on rehabilitation and alignment of the bones.

I have worked with clients who have been doing Pilates at some other studio three times a week for years, yet when I start working with them, they can't perform even the beginning abdominal exercises.

In my certification program at Ellie Herman Studios, I try to incorporate both fitness and rehabilitation when training my teachers, because I don't see the need to limit their approach to Pilates. A trainer with a deep understanding of Pilates that is coupled with a deep understanding of anatomy and alignment has the tools to help you heal from an injury and (depending on your individual needs and desires) also give you a great workout. Once trainers understand the Pilates method and how to break down the exercises to their most fundamental level, they can train almost anyone, no matter what the person's physical limitations or strengths may be.

Some trainers may spend an hour with you trying to get you to feel Neutral Spine and working on your breath. You won't even break a sweat. Other trainers may put you into contortionist positions before you're ready. Just ask your trainer to describe her approach before you begin, and communicate to your trainer exactly what you expect and desire from your workout. Don't settle for less. If you don't like your trainer, try another, because trainers vary immensely in their style, approach, and body knowledge. Don't give up on Pilates trainers until you've given them a good try!

Does the Studio Offer Group Classes on the Mat and/or the Equipment?

Group mat classes are one of the best ways to try out Pilates without a huge money commitment. Mat classes are usually less than $15 each and teach core strength and spinal flexibility. If you find that you love the Pilates mat work, then you can decide whether you're ready and willing to shell out money for private sessions to work on the equipment. Usually only the bigger studios offer group classes on the Pilates equipment, for the obvious reason that it takes space to have multiple pieces of the same equipment. If you can find group classes on the equipment, that's the most inexpensive way to try out the equipment and get a full-body Pilates workout. Most common are reformer classes and Pilates spring board classes, also sometimes called wall unit classes.

Is the Studio Fully Equipped?

Some small or independent studios may have only a reformer (see Chapter 15) and a mat. This doesn't necessarily mean it's a bad studio. I started out with just these two things, and everyone had a great time. But if you're curious about what the full Pilates system has to offer, try to find a studio that has at least a reformer, a cadillac, and a wunda chair.

Does the Studio Offer a Discount for a Class Series?

Most studios offer discounts if you buy five or more sessions at once. If this is the case, you can usually save between $5 and $15 per session. Ask about this offer before you sign up so that you don't spend more money than necessary.

How Much Is Too Much for a Pilates Session?

As this book goes to press, I charge $55 to $65 for a private session and $35 to $45 for a two-person class at my studios in San Francisco and Oakland. Group classes on the equipment range from $15 to $25, depending on the number of people in the class. A drop-in mat class costs between $10 and $15. You can use these prices as a guide for what to expect, although prices vary depending on the overhead of the studio and geography. I tend to be on the lower end of pricing in the Bay Area, so don't feel bad if you can't find prices in that range. But please don't pay more than $90 an hour unless you live in Beverly Hills or the Upper East Side of Manhattan, your Pilates teacher makes house calls, or you're working out with a master teacher.

Who Manages the Studio?

Find out whether the studio you're interested in is run by someone who actually knows Pilates. If it's a larger studio with many teachers, it's important that the person in charge really knows her stuff and maintains a standard of excellence.

Here's a horror story from my own experience. During a teacher training intensive workshop that I offered at my studio, a woman enrolled who was opening up a Pilates studio in a neighboring city. She proceeded to recruit half-trained instructors from the training program and hired them to work at her studio, against my screaming protestations. This woman was never certified in Pilates, and neither were her trainers. I have since heard that clients who went to this woman's studio have gotten injured and have had a negative Pilates experience.

Great Pilates studios and instructors

There are a lot of great teachers out there. For an international directory of Pilates instructors, call Balanced Body Inc. at 1-800-Pilates. It's on the Web at www.pilates.com.

If you're in the Bay Area, give my studios a call at 415-285-5808 (San Francisco) or 510-594-8507 (Oakland). I'm on the Web at www.ellie.net.

Here's a list of teachers and studios that I personally know are great:

✔ **Kathy Grant in New York City** (212-998-1983): Kathy Grant is a skinny eighty-something New Yorker, ex-Broadway dancer, and old-school Pilates teacher. In fact, she was one of Joe Pilates' original students. She's constantly making up whimsical and brilliant images to better describe to her students how to perform exercises to her exacting standards. She has healed many a dancer from many an injury. She has a small studio above the NYU dance department that houses, I believe, some of the oldest remaining pieces of Pilates equipment.

✔ **Cara Reeser in Denver** (carareeser@ earthlink.net): Cara is a devoted Pilates practitioner and healing artist. She has been studying for several years under Kathy Grant, one of the first generation of Pilates teachers, and has been able to share Kathy Grant's work nationally. Kathy basically healed Cara after a serious back injury, and Cara continued working with her for years after. Now Cara travels around the country giving workshops based on Kathy Grant's ideas. I recommend attending one if you have more than a fleeting interest in Pilates. In addition, she has a lovely little

studio in Denver, where she gives private lessons. Her studio, however, offers mat classes and semiprivate classes as well as private sessions.

✔ **Erica Essner in New York City** (essner@ eecop.org): Erica was certified by Ellie Herman Studios and also received extensive training from Jennifer Stacey in San Francisco. She is a professional dancer with her own company and a former massage therapist. Because of her extensive background in these various physical modalities, she has a great knowledge of the body that runs deeper than many Pilates instructors. She has a great New York attitude to boot.

✔ **The Pilates Center in Boulder** (www.thepilatescenter.com): The Pilates Center is one of the best places to get certified in the Pilates method. Many a great teacher has come out of the Boulder school. The studio also offers private, semiprivate, and group classes.

✔ **Centre Pilates de Paris** (www.centre pilates.com): Martine Curtis-Oakes and Laura Blackburn recently opened a studio in the heart of Paris. They have a great Web site with videos of cool Pilates moves; check it out!

✔ **Jelena Petrovic in Amsterdam** (jelenas light@hotmail.com): Jelena was certified by Ellie Herman Studios and has had lots of training from many other teachers. She is smart and spunky and has a beautiful British accent.

Chapter 22

Ten Ways to Complement Your Pilates Workout

. . . .

In This Chapter

▶ Improving your overall health

▶ Adding an aerobic element to your workout

. . . .

*T*his chapter gives you some ways to enhance your Pilates experience and enforce some of the concepts that you learn from Pilates. Pilates is great, but what you do when you're not doing Pilates is important, too.

Pilates does not become aerobic until you get to the advanced level. For your overall health, you need to have some aerobic element in your fitness regimen. Twenty to thirty minutes of aerobic exercise three times a week is the minimum you should be getting. Several of the suggestions in this chapter are about ways to get that aerobic workout.

Dancing

Whether it be ballet, modern, tap, or tango, dancing is a great way to incorporate the skills you learn in Pilates. Dance is like an even more flowing Pilates workout. Dance and Pilates are close sisters; they mutually feed and support each other.

If you're already a dancer, you'll immediately feel the benefits Pilates offers in the way of improving technique, balance, center control, and stamina.

Doing Yoga

If you're very tight, yoga is the most efficient way to increase your flexibility. Most yoga classes focus on opening up your body and increasing the range of motion in your spine, hips, and shoulders. Because yoga is so concerned with stretching out your muscles and joints, it's a great complement to Pilates.

Without a certain base amount of flexibility, you'll find many Pilates exercises quite difficult, and some impossible. Adding yoga to your routine will make you more limber so that you can get into Pilates positions more easily.

I think yoga teachers and students can all benefit from a few Pilates mat classes, and Pilates teachers and students can benefit from yoga. If you are already a yogi, you'll enjoy the extra focus on core strength and stabilization that you get in Pilates.

Many people come to me after being injured in yoga class. Unfortunately, many yoga teachers don't emphasize supporting extreme poses from the center. Use what you learn from your Pilates workout about alignment and deep abdominal engagement when you embark on a yoga class.

Eating Light

When you scoop your belly in, it helps if you don't have a heavy meal inside. Always eat light before a Pilates workout, and wait at least 2 hours after a meal before attempting to pull your navel to your spine. Eating light is generally a good idea anyway; go easy on cheeses, creamy sauces, fried foods, and large portions of meat. I recommend consuming lots of veggies, grains, fish, and soy products instead!

Getting a Massage

I find very few things more relaxing than a good massage. Massage can be one of the best and most efficient ways to address muscle tension and can be a great complement to Pilates because it relaxes tight and overworked muscles and helps bring balance back to the body. If you've never had a massage, I highly recommend finding a certified massage therapist and giving it a try, especially if you hold lots of tension in your neck and upper back. You may not like to be touched all over your body, but if you can get over that discomfort, you may end up with a new addiction.

Meditating

Meditation is a way for you to get grounded, become aware of your breath, and become more in touch with your body. Because both Pilates and meditation bring you back to your body and heighten your awareness in general, they are mutually beneficial.

There are many ways to meditate, and I can't say which is best for you. Experiment, and search the Web or read a book such as *Meditation For Dummies* by Stephan Bodian (Hungry Minds, Inc.) if you need more information.

Swimming

Swimming is a great complement to Pilates. It can be the aerobic component to your exercise regimen, and it's also nonimpact resistance exercise. The pool (or whatever body of water you're in) acts as your resistance as you stroke your arms and kick your legs. Because water creates resistance without impact, swimming builds long and lean muscles — just like Pilates. Also, you can apply your newfound body awareness and core strength to your swimming technique. You'll be pleasantly surprised by how much more power you have in your stroke when you work from the powerhouse!

Taking a Stretch Class

Yoga can be fairly extreme in terms of some of the poses asked of its students. If yoga is intimidating for you and you're very tight, try to find a stretch class. Regular attendance at an hour-long class stretch class increases your flexibility immensely and helps you to progress more quickly in the Pilates method.

Taking Hot Baths

Hot baths are great for all those who use their body. Sitting in a hot bath calms and relaxes the body and the mind and soothes aching muscles even more than taking a hot shower does. This is partly because you can lie down and bring yourself to a complete stop and partly because the heat makes you sweat and detoxifies your body. Try a hot bath, especially if you find yourself sore after you begin Pilates.

Using Aerobic Machines

If you belong to a gym, getting on an elliptical machine, stationary bicycle, or treadmill gives your fitness program the necessary aerobic component. Most large gyms have an assortment of aerobic equipment, so you can have enough variety in your workouts to keep you interested. Regular aerobic exercise helps your endurance in Pilates and in your everyday life.

Walking

Nietzsche said, "All truly great thoughts are conceived by walking." Even if you don't have any great thoughts while walking, you'll still probably enjoy it. I love walking because it's a nonimpact aerobic sport that allows your mind to wander and your thoughts to clear. Because Pilates teaches proper alignment, you can apply the concepts you learn in your Pilates exercises to your everyday gait. In addition, adding an aerobic component to your fitness regimen is important because Pilates generally isn't considered aerobic.

Index

• C •

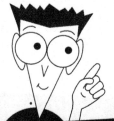
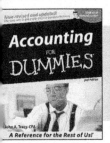
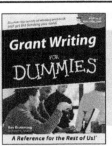
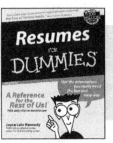
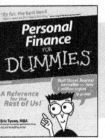
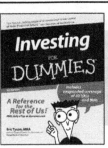
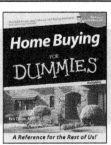
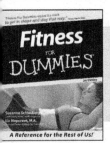
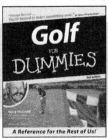
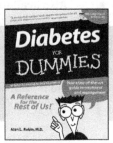
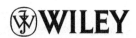

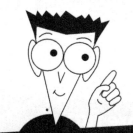

FOR DUMMIES®

A world of resources to help you grow

HOME, GARDEN & HOBBIES

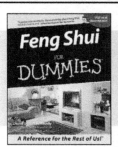

Feng Shui For Dummies
0-7645-5295-3

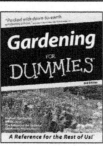

Gardening For Dummies
0-7645-5130-2

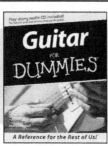

Guitar For Dummies
0-7645-5106-X

Also available:

Auto Repair For Dummies
(0-7645-5089-6)

Chess For Dummies
(0-7645-5003-9)

Home Maintenance For
Dummies
(0-7645-5215-5)

Organizing For Dummies
(0-7645-5300-3)

Piano For Dummies
(0-7645-5105-1)

Poker For Dummies
(0-7645-5232-5)

Quilting For Dummies
(0-7645-5118-3)

Rock Guitar For Dummies
(0-7645-5356-9)

Roses For Dummies
(0-7645-5202-3)

Sewing For Dummies
(0-7645-5137-X)

FOOD & WINE

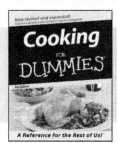

Cooking For Dummies
0-7645-5250-3

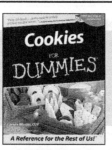

Cookies For Dummies
0-7645-5390-9

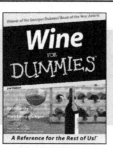

Wine For Dummies
0-7645-5114-0

Also available:

Bartending For Dummies
(0-7645-5051-9)

Chinese Cooking For
Dummies
(0-7645-5247-3)

Christmas Cooking For
Dummies
(0-7645-5407-7)

Diabetes Cookbook For
Dummies
(0-7645-5230-9)

Grilling For Dummies
(0-7645-5076-4)

Low-Fat Cooking For
Dummies
(0-7645-5035-7)

Slow Cookers For Dummies
(0-7645-5240-6)

TRAVEL

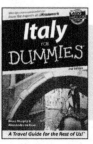

Italy For Dummies
0-7645-5453-0

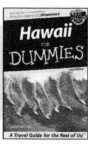

Hawaii For Dummies
0-7645-5438-7

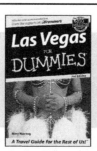

Las Vegas For Dummies
0-7645-5448-4

Also available:

America's National Parks For
Dummies
(0-7645-6204-5)

Caribbean For Dummies
(0-7645-5445-X)

Cruise Vacations For
Dummies 2003
(0-7645-5459-X)

Europe For Dummies
(0-7645-5456-5)

Ireland For Dummies
(0-7645-6199-5)

France For Dummies
(0-7645-6292-4)

London For Dummies
(0-7645-5416-6)

Mexico's Beach Resorts For
Dummies
(0-7645-6262-2)

Paris For Dummies
(0-7645-5494-8)

RV Vacations For Dummies
(0-7645-5443-3)

Walt Disney World & Orland
For Dummies
(0-7645-5444-1)

CPSIA information can be obtained
at www.ICGtesting.com
Printed in the USA
BVOW09s0216140917
494676BV00004B/7/P